You Can Beat Prostate Cancer

... And You Don't Need Surgery to Do it

New Edition

What Every Man and His Family Must Know
About Early Detection and Treatment

**This is the book the author wishes
had been available when he was
diagnosed with prostate cancer.**

By

Prostate Cancer Survivor

Robert J. Marckini

You Can Beat Prostate Cancer
And You Don't Need Surgery to Do It

By Robert J. Marckini

ISBN: 978-1-7342022-0-5

Comments/Endorsements

"It has been my privilege to call Bob Marckini a friend for a number of years. There are few lives more focused on helping others, particularly with prostate cancer, than Bob. But his message goes far beyond a cancer diagnosis and treatment options to a complete change in lifestyle and a new direction for each individual, from a state of fear to a journey of peace and gratitude. For two decades he has relentlessly pursued this vision of sharing information and understanding with many, through his best-selling book as well as endless phone calls, attendance at numerous meetings, and a monthly newsletter. There can be no question that Bob has altered the trajectory of countless lives, men and women, with this message of wholeness and health. It has been a privilege for Loma Linda University Health to partner with Bob on this journey of restoration."

~ Richard H. Hart, MD, DrPH, President, Loma Linda University
Health

~ ~ ~

"Bob Marckini's 2nd edition of You Can Beat Prostate Cancer is an outstanding guide for men who have been diagnosed with prostate cancer or, because of age or other factors, are at risk. Through an engaging personal narrative, he distills a plethora of information on the natural history of prostate cancer, countless patient experiences, and extensive published evidence into a few clear concepts that will aid prospective prostate cancer patients in navigating the difficult journey of choosing and completing a treatment strategy and as well as designing a healthy lifestyle to maximize long term treatment success and quality of life. The book is unique in that it provides both a thorough and rigorous investigation into the scientific evidence for specific management strategies as well as the authenticity of his own and others' lived experiences with various treatment options. All men concerned about prostate cancer should study this book and all physicians who treat prostate cancer should read this book and offer it to their patients."

~Nancy Price Mendenhall, MD, FASTRO, Professor, Dept. of
Radiation Oncology, Medical Director, Univ. of Florida Health
Proton Therapy Institute.

~ ~ ~

"You have just been told that you have prostate cancer. The "C" word. Do not panic. Most likely, there are multiple options that can lead to a great result and that's what makes prostate cancer decision-making so challenging. Bob Marckini again does a great job of walking patients through this complex decision-making process in the 2nd edition of his book which has been significantly updated. Not all of the available options for prostate cancer management are discussed with men by their doctors. Mr. Marckini does a fantastic job of exposing the reader to such options. If you have been diagnosed with prostate cancer, or know someone who has, you owe it to yourself, or them, to read this book."

~Sameer Keole, MD, Medical Director Proton Therapy, Mayo Clinic, Phoenix, AZ

~ ~ ~

"For men diagnosed with prostate cancer, Bob Marckini in this book clarifies from a patient's perspective why proton therapy is an ideal treatment option over surgery in order to preserve erections, eliminate incontinence, and prevent penile shortening. . . A must read for prostate cancer patients and their families."

~Steven J. Frank, MD, FACR, Professor and Executive Director, The UT MD Anderson Cancer Center Particle Therapy Institute

~ ~ ~

"As is true of many adult and pediatric cancers, there are [fortunately!] many options when it comes to treating prostate cancer and in my clinical experience, I routinely find that the most difficult decision patients face is which one to choose. Beginning with the publication of his first edition of "You Can Beat Prostate Cancer," and even more so new with his update, Bob Marckini provides a readable, factual guide for patients and their loved ones who are faced with this daunting but curable diagnosis, written in a style which is blessedly free of the jargon and acronyms which so often dominates the medical literature. It's an excellent resource which I recommend unequivocally"

~Carl J. Rossi MD, Medical Director, California Protons

~ ~ ~

"This book has EVERYTHING you need to know about prostate cancer, even if you are not a prostate cancer patient but have been touched by this disease in some way. By reading this book you will learn about how to deal with any serious illness and how to master your own health management. This new edition summarizes the feedback from many scientists, patients and from the readership of Bob Marckini's "*BOB Tales* Monthly Newsletter" during the past 20 years. This great book is an incredible resource for anyone seeking knowledge about serious health problems and a comprehensive manual on how to manage through them. The book is a "must read" and should be an important asset in everybody's library."

~Arnd Hallmeyer, MD, PhD, DSc, Prostate Cancer Survivor, Berlin, Germany

~ ~ ~

"I recommend this book to every patient or family member affected by an elevated PSA or a diagnosis of prostate cancer. In medicine, we are taught that invasive procedures should only be done if less intrusive tests or

iv

interventions are not effective or available. This updated book accurately captures critical information on less invasive (and more precise) methods of diagnosis and treatment of prostate cancer. Although prostate removal may be right for some men, it should never be accepted by a patient until they have fully considered and vetted less-invasive alternatives such as modern active surveillance or proton therapy. Thank you Bob (and Deb) for your long-term commitment to sharing this information with the world!"

~J. Ben Wilkinson, MD, FACRO, Radiation Oncologist

~ ~ ~

"For any patient faced with the diagnosis of prostate cancer, there will be fear and anxiety. Most men will do well if they are educated on the nature and status of their disease. In easy to read language, Robert Marckini's book does an excellent job of informing patients on their prostate cancer diagnosis, treatment options, life after treatment, and much more. "You Can Beat Prostate Cancer" is a practical and comprehensive guide for men at risk for prostate cancer or for men recently diagnosed with the disease. This is a book that every prostate cancer patient should read before making a decision on treatment or surveillance."

~Joseph J. Busch Jr. MD Oncological Radiologist, Busch Center
Kathy Busch BS, RT (N) (MR), (CT), CNMT (PET)

~ ~ ~

"There is a reason that Bob Marckini's book has been a top seller for over 10 years. This book is an island of current and pertinent information with rational and deductive thinking in a sea of limitless prostate cancer information and misinformation. I highly recommend that men diagnosed with or at risk for prostate cancer read and share with their family this easy to understand book."

~Les Yonemoto, MD, MBA, CPE, DABR

~ ~ ~

"This book chronicles Bob's research into the treatment options he was presented with, discusses the pros and cons of those and other available treatments, his decision-making process, treatment, and experiences since. This second edition remains a must-read for any man (or his partner) facing a diagnosis of prostate cancer. Despite the fact that proton therapy has been around for many years, most providers know very little about it. It often falls on the patient to find and explore this option. In this edition, he has added helpful sections on current research, staying healthy after cancer and adding more personal stories from men who have been treated with protons. This book is a great place to start your research, as Bob has done much of the homework for you."

~Carolyn Vachani, RN, MSN, AOCN, OncoLink, Penn Medicine,
Abramson Cancer Center, Managing Editor,
cvachani@oncolink.org, 215-901-4807, www.oncolink.org

"It is with great pleasure that I give my highest endorsement to the second edition of Bob Marckini's book on prostate cancer diagnosis and treatment. I am a senior cancer researcher and academic medical educator and have many publications in cancer biology. For over thirty years I taught medical students and physicians in training. I am also a proton therapy prostate cancer survivor, having had proton therapy treatment in 2002. All of this means that I have a unique perspective about this book. The book is an informative guide for patients who have, or want to learn about prostate cancer, and treatment options. It is comprehensive, clearly written, and shows an unbelievable amount of thoughtfulness by the author. When you read this book, you will become extremely well informed on the topic. It will help you understand your diagnosis, and sort through all the treatment options. It can also help you to make the right decisions for your future. Bob truly wants to help men with prostate cancer to make the best-informed choices for their future. He has accomplished this, and we are the beneficiaries of his compassionate efforts. Thanks, Bob, for all your hard work and dedication."

~H. Terry Wepsic, MD, Professor Emeritus of Pathology,
University of California, Irvine, CA, Research Professor, Long
Beach VA Healthcare System, Long Beach, CA

~ ~ ~

"You Can Beat Prostate Cancer" helps expose the confusion and misinformation surrounding the term prostate cancer and is an important public health resource for any man receiving this sorry label. Bob Marckini's personal journey, insights and challenges to so-called conventional wisdom also lead to his development of an equally amazing prostate cancer support group that helps men understand their particular diagnosis before they make reckless decisions and are robbed of health."

~Bert Vorstman MD, MS, FAAP, FRACS, FACS, Board Certified
Urologist (Retired)

~ ~ ~

"The second edition of this book represents the most objective, comprehensive, authoritative and yet layperson-friendly synopsis of everything a newly diagnosed prostate cancer victim needs to know about prostate cancer prevention, diagnosis and treatment options. Armed with this information, gleaned by Bob Marckini over many years, the reader should be able to make an informed decision whether to be treated and if so by what mode of treatment. Many myths about proton therapy are dispelled and many risk factors associated with other treatment options are brought to light. This book will save lives and will greatly improve the quality of life for many prostate cancer victims!"

~Patrick Greany, PhD retired USDA Research Entomologist and
Courtesy Professor, University of Florida.

"Prostate cancer patients and their loved ones face a bewildering choice of treatment options. Bob Marckini draws on his 20 years of experience as prostate cancer survivor and nationally recognized patient advocate to make a compelling, well balanced case for prostate cancer patients to consider proton therapy for their treatment."

~John B. Frick, Managing Director, Chisholm Advisors

~ ~ ~

"In March of 2008 at my annual physical, my PSA jumped up. Fortunately for me, a close friend, who had been diagnosed with prostate cancer the previous year, had a copy of Bob Marckini's first book and gave it to me. After reading it, I flew up to visit Bob Marckini. How lucky can you get? After talking with Bob, I went to Loma Linda University Cancer Center for proton treatment. Since my wonderful treatment experience with no cancer recurrence and no impotence, incontinence or other side effects after 12 years, I have devoted my life to helping those who are faced with prostate cancer treatment options. Reading Bob's book was one of the single most important things I've done in my life."

~Charles A. Smithgall III, Former Chairman and CEO of SEI
Aaron's, Inc.

~ ~ ~

"Bob Marckini has done a wonderful job in updating and expanding the scope of this book, capturing important advances in screening, diagnosis, staging and treatment options for prostate cancer therapies. In regards to proton therapy, important advances are described such as utilization of pencil beam scanning which enables the delivery of IMPT- Intensity Modulated Proton Therapy. Over the years, I worked with all 3 modalities of proton therapy: Double scatter, Uniform scanning and IMPT. Use of IMPT has been revolutionary allowing larger treatment fields such those to treat pelvic lymph nodes in high risk prostate cancer. Another advancement in our field also referenced in this book is the utilization of rectal spacer (SpaceOAR) which displaces the rectum away from the prostate to further reduce rectal exposure to high doses of radiation. As a pioneer adopter of rectal spacer in proton therapy, I treated the first patients worldwide with this combination in April of 2015 following FDA clearance. In my experience of well over 500 patients treated with protons and rectal spacer, I can attest to excellent treatment tolerance, significant reductions in rectal dose exposure and treatment related gastro-intestinal side-effects."

~Marcio Fagundes, MD, Medical Director – Radiation Oncology
Department, Miami Cancer Institute

~ ~ ~

"Before retiring in late 2019, I was Vice President of Professional Education at Augmenix, which was purchased by Boston Scientific in October of 2018. My duties focused on training leading physicians around the world. During that time, I had the opportunity to meet Bob Marckini and read the first edition of his book. I also witnessed the influence of his ministry promoting prostate cancer awareness, prevention and treatment, and tending to the 10,000 members of the prostate cancer support group he founded. Bob's knowledge and intellectual curiosity on this subject is second to none, witnessed at many major meetings dealing with promoting awareness and understanding prostate cancer. I consider his second edition to be the most comprehensive, complete treatment of the subject today, and a must read for anyone diagnosed with prostate cancer or at risk for the disease."

~Tom Guest, Johnson and Johnson, Vice President of Professional Education, Augmenix/Boston Scientific

~ ~ ~

"If you've been diagnosed with prostate cancer, don't be rushed into deciding what to do about it. This is a slow-growing disease. You have time to make what will be one of the most important decisions of your life. You may need "definitive treatment" – a euphemism for surgery or radiation that will change the quality of your life forever. Or you may need to do nothing at all but monitor your disease, an approach known as active surveillance. Robert J. Marckini was diagnosed with prostate cancer 20 years ago. He made a decision to undergo proton therapy, a noninvasive approach that has received scant attention. Marckini is an advocate for proton therapy, but thoroughly covers the many other options you may consider on your personal cancer journey. Get second opinions from doctors but prepare yourself by reading the new edition of Marckini's "You Can Bear Prostate Cancer." This book will serve as your guide as you prepare for those second and third opinions from physicians and make your final decision."

~Howard Wolinsky, nine years on active surveillance for low-risk prostate cancer and author of "A Patient's Journey" column for MedPageToday.com

~ ~ ~

"Marckini has produced an exceptional work in sharing the trauma and the resulting journey associated with hearing the words, "you have cancer!" In a warm and convincing manner, he conveys his personal search for a 21st Century non-invasive treatment modality for his disease. His journey ends in finding hope, healing, health, happiness and wholeness. It is a must read for anyone confronted with cancer."

~J. Lynn Martell, DMin, Director of Special Services Loma Linda University Medical Center (Retired)

"Whoever survives a test, whatever it may be, must tell the story. That is his duty." – Elie Wiesel

To my wife, Pauline,
our two children, Susie and Deb,
my son in law Mark,
and my granddaughter, Gemma,
for their love and support.

x

Forward

Bert Vorstman, BSc, MD, MS, FAAP, FRACS, FACS is a Board-Certified Urological Surgeon. He recently wrote an important article, titled, "Is Robotic Prostate Cancer Surgery Bad Health Advice." It should be required reading for anyone with rising PSA, or who has recently been diagnosed with prostate cancer. This article appeared in Urology Web and can be found at https://urologyweb.com/is-robotic-prostate-cancer-surgery-bad-health-advice/

Near the beginning of the article, Dr. Vorstman wrote a paragraph on "Receiving a Prostate Cancer Diagnosis," which states:

Receiving a prostate cancer diagnosis can bring you to your knees. *In total disbelief you may feel terror, confused, vulnerable and desperate. It's difficult to think about anything else. You just don't know where to begin, who to turn to, or who you can trust. Slowly, you begin your information gathering only to find out that there is no emergency, no standard way of managing your particular diagnosis, little time to ask questions, and perhaps pressured by scare tactics to choose a course of action. At every turn there is a different story. Shockingly, even the prostate cancer support groups and online forums can't always be trusted. Before long, you learn that the prostate cancer arena is filled with misconceptions, assumptions, and distortions. Dissatisfied and frustrated, you just want to get it all behind you, but take your time and get a second opinion regarding your biopsy results.* ***Ultimately however, you will have to make a difficult decision based upon what type of prostate cancer you have, whether or not it seems contained and what you believe is right for you. Still, you're left with a feeling that the acceptable is really unacceptable.***

When I read that paragraph, I thought, "Dr. Vorstman must have read the first edition of my book!" And while I don't agree with every point made in this important article, I do agree with most of what he has to say, beginning with the paragraph above.

The journey you are about to begin is a tough one, but a manageable one. If you go about it thoughtfully, systematically and with an open mind, you will make the right decision for dealing with your diagnosis; the right decision for your family; and most importantly, the right decision for *yourself.*

Preface

My older brother had always been the strong one in the family. After my father died, Gene, then 45, became the patriarch. He took Dad's place as the family leader and he was good at it. Highly educated, well read, and in excellent physical condition, Gene, in his 6-foot 1-inch frame, became the one everybody turned to for advice and counsel.

Nineteen years later, in 1998, I was standing in the recovery room of a major Boston hospital when they wheeled Gene in from surgery. He had been diagnosed with prostate cancer three months earlier and had undergone a radical prostatectomy (surgical removal of the prostate) on his physician's advice.

What I wasn't prepared for was how serious the surgery was, how deep the surgeon's scalpel had to cut, and how careful they had to be to spare critical nerves and blood vessels in order to give him the best chance of retaining his sexual potency and bladder control. I also hadn't realized how much blood he would lose – six pints in all.

There, lying on the hospital gurney was someone I barely recognized. His face was ashen; his eyes hollow. Attached to his body were numerous tubes, drains, IV's, a Foley catheter for urine drainage, an oxygen mask, and electronic monitors. My older brother, who four hours earlier was the picture of health, appeared to be inches away from death.

This experience had a profound impact on me. I had never seen my big brother in such a weakened and vulnerable condition. His situation was also of particular interest because my PSA was elevated, and I was scheduled for a prostate biopsy the following week. Since both my father and brother were prostate cancer victims, my chances of being diagnosed with the same disease were high.

I made a promise to myself in the recovery room that day:

"If I'm ever diagnosed with prostate cancer, I will do exhaustive research to determine if there is a reasonable alternative to surgery."

Two years and three biopsies later, I was diagnosed, and I began my research.

I found four major treatment options for prostate cancer, and one essentially unknown alternative. The biggest surprise came when I discovered that the "unknown" option was quite authentic; it was painless; it involved no invasive surgery; and the success rate on thousands of patients treated over many years was comparable to "the gold standard," surgery. I also discovered that with this treatment there were minimal, if any, long-term side effects; and it was covered by Medicare and most private medical insurance providers. Yet most people, patients and doctors were not aware of its existence.

After completing my research, which included reading all available technical literature on and off the Web, and interviewing dozens of prostate cancer patients, I decided to have proton beam therapy at Loma Linda University Cancer Center in Loma Linda, California. This decision changed my life.

The baby boomer generation – currently ages 56 – 76 – is in the prime prostate cancer age range; and Generation X men – ages 40 – 55 aren't far behind. One of six men in each group will be diagnosed with prostate cancer. How will they deal with this?

Most will choose surgery for prostate removal on their urologist's recommendation. Yet most don't need a radical prostatectomy. They can be treated by non-invasive options, which can provide comparable cure rates, carry far fewer risks than surgery and preserve their quality of life.

One of these non-invasive options is a state-of-the-art, painless procedure known as proton therapy. The problem is very few people have even heard of this treatment. They soon will, as dozens of medical centers all over the world are making the multi-million-dollar capital investment in this extraordinary technology.

This book is my story. It takes you from the horror of my prostate cancer diagnosis, through several anxious months of research, decision-making, treatment and life after treatment.

This book is also a guide for newly diagnosed men and their families. It's intended to help them navigate through the myriad of technical details, treatment options, medical terminology, and the wide range of emotions that accompany this diagnosis and journey.

This is the book I wish had been available to me when I was diagnosed with prostate cancer on August 10, 2000.

Introduction

If you've recently been diagnosed with prostate cancer you're probably frightened. I was. You may also be confused. Most of us aren't prepared for this diagnosis. I had no symptoms. I was a physically fit 57-year-old non-smoker who ran three miles a day, ate a healthy diet and felt great.

And then the doctor told me I had prostate cancer. What do I do now? Do I put myself in my doctor's hands? Or, do I find out everything I can about this disease, evaluate *all* the options, interview anyone/everyone who can provide substantive information, and *then* decide what's best for *me*? Thank God I chose the latter option.

This is a true story of my diagnosis, my research into the many treatment options, my decision and the outcome. It's also a summary of all the important things I learned along the way; things I didn't find in any of the books or articles I read about prostate cancer treatment; things I wish I had known from the start.

I make no claim that this is a complete and objective review of all prostate cancer treatment options. After hundreds of hours of research, I chose – what was then – a relatively new approach called proton therapy. I admit I'm partial to this treatment modality. Why? Because it's non-invasive; it's painless; and it results in minimal to no side effects. But mostly – because it works.

I strongly feel that anyone with early – mid – or advanced stage prostate cancer, without metastasis – i.e. localized disease – should seriously consider this treatment, and I'll explain why in this book. However, I must point out – I'm not a doctor; I don't work in the medical field; and what is presented in this book is purely my opinion. It is, however, an opinion based on my initial research, analysis, interviews with hundreds of prostate cancer patients including many physician-patients and – in this second edition – 19 additional years of research and reflection.

My decision to have proton therapy changed my life so dramatically that I feel compelled to tell the world my story. Whether or not you choose proton therapy as your prostate cancer treatment, you'll find this book helpful in guiding you through the complexities of the journey you're about to begin.

Other Books on Prostate Cancer are Written by Doctors

In my research I discovered, not to my surprise, that the hundreds of prostate cancer books available were typically authored by doctors. This, of course, gives the reader comfort in knowing that the claims made in the book are made by credentialed medical professionals. However, the books are often highly technical in nature and even with my engineering background, I had difficulty understanding some of the concepts. Also evident in my reading was the fact that each author was inclined to "steer" the patient in the direction of his or her specialty. How objectively can a urologist – who is fundamentally a surgeon – write about radiation; a radiation oncologist – write about surgery; or a brachytherapist – write about cryoablation?

The question I kept asking myself in the early stage of my journey was, "Whom can I go to, to find the best course of action for Bob Marckini?" After a while, the answer became very clear – *I* had to do the work and *I* had to provide the answers.

So, why should you pay any attention to a book written about prostate cancer treatment by a non-medical person? It's simple. Who better to tell you about such an important experience and decision-making process than one who's been on the receiving end; one who went through it himself? Who better can share with you the terror of hearing the news – "you have prostate cancer" – and then tell you the story of how to deal with the emotions, the uncertainty, the ambiguity, and the unknowns connected with understanding this dreaded disease, and then making a life-changing treatment decision?

Amazon lists more than 3,000 books on the subject of prostate cancer diagnosis and treatment. Most of them are well written. They explain in great detail the technology and statistics from a medical professional's point of view. This book is intended to approach the subject of prostate cancer from the *patient's* point of view. Certainly, any claims made in this book can be easily verified by talking with professionals in the field, by searching the Internet or by talking with former patients.

As I look back on my hundreds of hours of research, the interviews I conducted, and the people I met during treatment, I'm struck by the fact that the vast majority of men who elected proton therapy as their treatment option had several things in common. They were highly educated, technical or analytical people who took charge of their treatment and were able to research, analyze, digest and understand the technical details connected with proton therapy. These men were doctors, lawyers, college professors, engineers, scientists, CEOs, physicists, and other professionals who were comfortable wallowing in technical detail and data.

But these are not the only kind of men who develop prostate cancer. What about the store clerks, policemen, postmen, janitors, plumbers, taxi drivers, and other men in our society who aren't particularly technical or analytical by nature? What do they do when they're diagnosed with prostate cancer?

I found that most men simply put their treatment decision in the hands of their local doctors. While this may not be the *worst* thing to do, it was not for me. And, I learned in my journey that in many cases, turning this decision over to your primary care physician or your urologist is not in your best interest.

The deeper I dug into the various treatment options, the more I realized how important it was for me to take charge of my own treatment decision. In my research, I found that treating prostate cancer is not like fixing a broken bone, stitching a cut, bypassing a clogged artery or even treating other types of cancer. In these cases the treatment choices are usually quite clear and obvious.

With prostate cancer, however, a patient's options are many, and they are extremely disparate: Open surgery, robotic surgery, intensity modulated radiation therapy (IMRT), brachytherapy, cyberknife, thomotherapy, rapidArc, stereotatactic body radiation therapy (SBRT), calypso, proton therapy, hypofractionated radiation therapy, hormonal therapy, immunotherapy, cryotherapy, high intensity focused ultrasound (HIFU), focal laser ablation (FLA), and so on. With a list like this, it's easy for both physicians and patients to be confused. The challenge of choosing a prostate cancer treatment option is escalated when adding to the equation the patient's age and comorbidities (i.e. other chronic medical conditions).

How does one navigate through these treatment options and make an intelligent choice?

A Word about How to Use This Book

This book is written for men and women. Women often play a key role in the research and treatment decision-making process for their loved ones. You'll also find the book written in laymen's language. Highly technical terminology and jargon are avoided as much as possible.

In reviewing prostate cancer treatment options for example, I've attempted to cover the most important points in summary form and with few technical details. Excellent resources (books, Internet, etc.) are available to the reader for a more in-depth treatment of these subjects. Many of them were references for this work and are listed in the appendix. I've found that most people are not interested in the technical details, just the cold, hard facts.

Information presented here will be helpful to men who have recently been diagnosed with prostate cancer, men who have rising PSA, and men who are at higher risk for prostate cancer due to family history or other factors. Men already treated for prostate cancer, who are experiencing a recurrence, will also find this book useful.

This book is also written for healthy men, those who take their health seriously, are proactive in managing their wellness, and aren't waiting for the classical mid-to-late-stage physical symptoms of prostate cancer to show up before taking action.

You can either read this book front to back or read selected chapters for information or to answer specific questions. Chapters can be read out of order and still provide continuity and value to the reader. You will also notice that I intentionally repeat key points in this book for the sake of emphasis.

Helpful hints are found throughout the book as a way of highlighting key points. They are shown in bold print and italics.

One gentleman who read the first edition of my book had been told he had cancer and was scheduled for surgery. He followed one of my suggestions and got a second opinion on his biopsy slides from one of the premier pathology labs listed in the appendix. He discovered he didn't have prostate cancer at all. This and many other important, real-life stories are shared in this second edition.

Name Changes

Some of the names used in the book were changed to protect the individual's privacy. The people and situations described are all real, however.

Don't Skip the Appendix

Readers often pay little or no attention to the appendix in books. There is much valuable information presented in the appendix of this book, and I encourage you to spend some time there. In addition to a glossary of important terms, a list of proton centers within the U.S., a bibliography of important books and published articles, helpful prostate cancer websites, and premier pathology labs for a second opinion on your biopsy slides, there is an especially valuable resource in the appendix: Real-life stories written by former proton patients describing their prostate cancer journeys. I strongly recommend that you read the 24 testimonials. The stories are compelling.

Two Most Important Messages

Numerous points are made throughout this book that, hopefully, will aid you in your effort to prevent, treat, or otherwise deal with prostate cancer.

The two most important messages I hope you get from this book are 1) early detection greatly improves your chance for disease-free survival, and 2) you can and should take control of your treatment decision. If you get nothing more out of this book than a clearer understanding of these key points, your time and money will have been well spent.

One Last Point

If you are seriously considering surgery, skip to Chapter 6 and read the advantages and *especially* the disadvantages of having a radical prostatectomy, either open or robotic procedures.

NO MEDICAL ADVICE: Material appearing here represents opinions offered by non-medically trained laypersons. Comments shown here should NEVER be interpreted as specific medical advice and must be used only as background information when consulting with a qualified medical professional.

CONTENTS

APPENDIX

CHAPTER 1

Prostate Cancer – The Basics

"You will hear a lot of men who have been diagnosed with prostate cancer say they never had a symptom, never felt anything. That's because the most common symptom is no symptom at all." – *Sidney Poitier*

Prostate Cancer is on the Rise

All forms of cancer are on the rise. According to Karol Sikora, former chief of the World Health Organization Cancer Program, cancer rates are predicted to double over the next 20 years. The number of new cases of cancer is expected to increase from 10 million per year to 20 million per year, and the number of deaths will increase from 6 million to 12 million. In the U.S. alone, the *Cancer Journal for Clinicians* (Cancer J Clin 2016;66:7-3) tells us that about 1.7 million men and women would be diagnosed with cancer (all types) in 2016 and close to 600,000 would die from the disease.

What do we know about prostate cancer? We know that every 14 minutes a man dies of prostate cancer in the U.S. If you know a dozen men, two of them will be diagnosed with prostate cancer in their lifetime. In the first edition of this book, published in 2006, I reported:

"More than 200,000 cases will be diagnosed in the U.S. this year." The prostate cancer diagnosis rate is increasing 10 percent a year due to increased awareness and improved diagnostic techniques.

Since then, these numbers have dropped dramatically, but not because prostate cancer is going away. Rather, the diagnostic rate dropped because the United States Preventive Service Task Force

(USPSTF) took a position in 2012 recommending strongly against PSA testing. They took this action ostensibly because men diagnosed with early stage disease were being "over-treated" for prostate cancer and harmed by the treatment. Their position was that most of these men with early stage disease would never die from prostate cancer, but would suffer the life-changing consequences of urinary and sexual side effects from the major treatment options.

What the USPSTF failed to realize was that the problem was not "over-diagnosing" patients, it was "over-treating" patients. Many men with early stage disease could easily follow their disease using active surveillance (explained later) rather than choose one of the major treatment options that can alter the quality of their lives.

The result of the USPSTF's misguided action was a temporary reduction in the number of prostate cancer diagnoses in the U.S., but an increase in the number of missed diagnoses of more advanced cancers.

The USPSTF has since modified its stance on PSA testing, and as expected, the number of new cases is, once again, on the rise.

Black Men Most Vulnerable

Black men in the U.S. are 2.5 times more likely to die of prostate cancer compared to white men. Yet, the screening guidelines for black men are based primarily on studies of *white* men according to a recent Harvard University News & Research article titled, *Filling a Research Gap.*

The Harvard study reported that midlife PSA screening of black men can strongly predict total and aggressive prostate cancer many years into the future. Clearly, black men should be screened earlier in life than white men, yet this subject is not getting the attention it deserves.

Prostate cancer is the second-leading cause of cancer death for men, second only to lung cancer. According to the Cancer Group Institute, prostate cancer kills about 30,000 men each year in the U.S. alone. *Vanguard Health (2017)* reports that, globally, approximately 1.1 million men are diagnosed with prostate cancer and more than 300,000 will die of the disease.

No One is Immune

Prostate cancer has affected some notable people including actors Robert De Niro, Roger Moore, Ryan O'Neal, Sidney Poitier, Charlton Heston and Ben Stiller, Gov. Jerry Brown, Secretary of State John Kerry, Mayor Rudi Giuliani, Harry Belafonte, Warren Buffett, Sens. Robert Dole and Jesse Helms, Gens. Norman Schwarzkopf and Colin Powell, Nelson Mandela, sports figures Ken Venturi, Arnold Palmer, Ken Griffey Sr. and Joe Torre, just to name a few.

We hear about these high-profile men who have gone public with their diagnoses. But what about everyday men like your barber, your plumber, your minister or priest, the trash collector, the postman, your father-in-law, your brother, and yes – even you? All are at risk of being diagnosed with prostate cancer.

We know that if you are Black, North American, or Northwestern European, your prostate cancer risk is higher than for other groups. We also know that if close relatives have been diagnosed with prostate cancer your chances of being diagnosed increase dramatically (more on that later).

What can you do about this? Can prostate cancer be prevented? How is prostate cancer diagnosed? If you have it, can it be cured? What about side effects and quality of life after treatment? What's the best treatment option? All these important questions will be addressed and answered in this book.

Prevention

Genetics: Little is known about the causes of prostate cancer. We know that your chances of having prostate cancer are greater if your father or brother has had the disease. Recent studies have identified genes that seem to play a role in this arena. Short of choosing different relatives, there is nothing you can do about the heredity component.

Diet: Many studies indicate that diet is a contributing factor. Reports from Harvard University have shown that Western diets, including those with high levels of fat from red meat and whole dairy products, increase your risk. Higher-than-average intakes of sugar, alcohol or total calories are also attributed to increased risk. Affluent

3

industrial societies that consume large amounts of refined flour also have higher prostate cancer incidence.

Other studies show that eating certain vegetables, fish, cereals and other whole-grain products seem to reduce the risk of prostate cancer. Fruits, nuts and seeds also appear to reduce the risk of prostate cancer, yet the reasons have not been determined. One study proposed the benefits come from higher levels of boron in these foods.

Investigators at the American Association of Cancer Researchers recently reported that a natural substance found in common fruits and vegetables significantly reduced the production of a key protein in hormone-dependent forms of prostate cancer.

One study in Italy compared 10,149 patients who were diagnosed with cancer between 1983 and 1996, to 7,990 patients who were hospitalized for non-malignant diseases. The results showed significant evidence that the men who ate larger quantities of whole grain foods had a 20 percent *lower* risk of developing prostate cancer.

Vegetable fats may reduce risk. A Canadian study involving 1,025 men found that those who consumed the most vegetable fats were 60 to 67 percent less likely to develop prostate cancer. Cruciferous vegetables, such as broccoli, cabbage and Brussels sprouts seem to be particularly beneficial.

Tomatoes/Lycopene: A Loma Linda University study linked higher levels of tomato consumption to protection against prostate cancer. Higher levels of lycopene in the blood are associated with lower prostate cancer rates. A Harvard University study identified tomatoes as one of the most "productive" vegetables you can have in your diet. This has been confirmed in other studies as well.

Lycopene, an antioxidant, is the substance that gives tomatoes their red color. Very simply, lycopene helps prevent cells in the body from "rusting." In doing so, lycopene helps block the uncontrolled multiplication of cancer cells. If you cannot eat at least 10 tomato servings a week, preferably *cooked* tomatoes, you should consider taking lycopene capsule supplements.

Asians: Asians are less likely to develop prostate cancer than their Western counterparts. Some experts feel this is due to the Asian diet, which is high in soy products such as tofu, soy milk, and miso. Asians also drink large quantities of tea. One study raises the possibility that there are compounds in tea that fight prostate cancer.

4

Vitamin D: Finally, vitamin D in reasonable doses has been shown to lower the likelihood of developing prostate cancer in some men.

Where I Fit In: Since my father had developed prostate cancer many years ago, I figured I needed all these things. My diet was already healthy. Red meat was something I consumed about once a month. Fish and chicken (skin removed) were a regular part of my diet. My wife always served lots of fresh vegetables at mealtime. I consumed very little sugar or alcohol. Multiple vitamins and whole-grain foods have been a part of my diet for years. I had done my homework, so lycopene and higher doses of vitamin D were already a part of my morning vitamin ritual.

Except for choosing different parents, I felt I had done almost everything possible to minimize my chances of getting this disease. Nevertheless, I developed prostate cancer, as did my older brother. I concluded that there must be something to this heredity thing!

Based on my research, and discussions with patients, physicians (internists, urologists and oncologists), and health educators, I learned that as men get older, we should be taking certain vitamins and supplements daily.

Prevention Summary: No one can tell you exactly what to do to prevent prostate cancer. What *can* be said, however, is that something, over which we have no control – heredity – does play an important role. It can also be said that you may be able to significantly reduce your chances of developing prostate cancer if you eat a diet low in animal fat, sugars, and alcohol, along with fish, fruits, vegetables, whole-grain foods, nuts, and certain supplements. I will elaborate on this in later chapters.

What is a Prostate?

The prostate is a walnut-sized gland located between the base of the penis and the bladder. The urethra, a tube that carries urine from the bladder to the penis, passes through the center of the prostate. The function of the prostate is to produce part of the fluid that makes up the semen. During the process of ejaculation, the prostate contracts and forces fluid into the urethra along with the seminal vesicles, which surround the prostate. Sperm ejected from the testes also enters the urethra and mixes with the seminal fluids during orgasm.

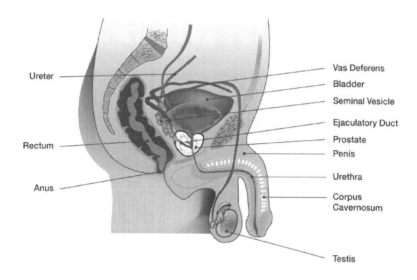

As men grow older, it's common for the prostate to become enlarged. As the prostate grows there is a tendency for it to begin to restrict, or pinch-off, the urethra. This is a common cause of men's inability to completely empty the bladder. Unfortunately for many men, this creates the need to make frequent trips to the bathroom.

There are several diseases of the prostate. The three most common are prostatitis, BPH and prostate cancer.

Prostatitis

Prostatitis is a common infection of the prostate gland. The cause is not known. Some experts believe that prostatitis is an autoimmune problem. Others feel that prostatitis is a combination of several infections or diseases. Acute prostatitis with fever is usually caused by a bacterial infection. Yet other prostatitis symptoms have nothing to do with bacterial infection. Antibiotics are often prescribed for prostatitis and have proven to be effective.

BPH

BPH (Benign Prostatic Hyperplasia) is the most common non-cancer cause of prostate enlargement. By age 60, fully half the male population will develop BPH. That number increases to 90 percent by age 86.

There are several treatment options for BPH. These include watchful waiting, medical therapy, balloon dilation, stents, and surgery. Every year in the U.S., approximately 300,000 surgeries are performed to relieve the symptoms of BPH.

The American Urological Association (AUA) has prepared a series of questions to help determine the presence of BPH. By answering these seven questions about the severity of symptoms, it is possible to define whether the symptoms are mild (0-7 points), moderate (8-19 points) or severe (20-35 points):

Questions to be answered: Over the past month . . .	Not at all	Less than 1 time in 5	Less than ½ the time	About ½ the time	More than ½ the time	Al-most always
1. How often have you had a sensation of not emptying your bladder completely after you finished urinating?	0	1	2	3	4	5
2. How often have you had to urinate again less than 2 hours after you finished urinating?	0	1	2	3	4	5
3. How often have you found you stopped and started again several times when you urinated?	0	1	2	3	4	5
4. How often have you found it difficult to postpone urination?	0	1	2	3	4	5
5. How often have you had a weak urinary stream?	0	1	2	3	4	5
6. How often have you had to push or strain to begin urination?	0	1	2	3	4	5
7. How many times did you most typically get up to urinate from the time you went to bed at night until the time you got up in the morning?	0	1	2	3	4	5

Sum of 7 circled numbers (AUA Symptom Score): _____

Prostate Cancer

Prostate cancer is clearly the most serious disease of the prostate. As mentioned earlier, it's the second-leading cause of cancer death in men, surpassed only by lung cancer. Yet with early detection this disease is highly curable.

Prostate cancer develops from cells in the prostate gland. The most common cancer of the prostate is *adenocarcinoma*. Generally, this cancer is slow growing. New detection techniques are allowing doctors to find it in the early stages. When this happens, the chances of a cure are very good. As men grow older and die of diseases other than prostate cancer, autopsies often reveal the presence of prostate cancer. It's often said that most men will not die *of* prostate cancer, but they will die *with* it.

According to WebMD, almost all men with prostate cancer will survive more than five years after diagnosis. About 5 percent of newly diagnosed men have more advanced prostate cancer, some with metastasis (spread to other parts of the body). About one-third of these men will survive for five years after diagnosis – a good case for early detection. Overall, the 10-year survival rate for prostate cancer is 91 percent and at 15 years that rate falls to 76 percent.

Early Detection

Unfortunately, the physical symptoms of prostate cancer often arrive after the cancer has had the opportunity to grow and spread beyond the prostate gland. This makes treatment more difficult, and the success rate lower – all the more reason for routine testing to identify the presence of the disease at the earliest possible stage.

The importance of early detection cannot be overemphasized. Here's a summary of facts from the American Cancer Society, the National Prostate Cancer Coalition and the Centers for Disease Control and Prevention (CDC):

Approximate number of prostate-cancer deaths in U.S. in 2017	28,000
Approximate number of new cases each year	200,000
Lifetime risk of developing prostate cancer among American men	1 in 6
Five-year survival rate for men with early stage disease	100%
Five-year survival rate for men whose prostate cancer has spread to distant parts of the body at diagnosis	31%

I suspect that with improvements in detection and treatment in recent years, survival rates will continue to improve. And the value of early detection is obvious by these numbers. Early stage prostate cancer is almost always confined to the gland or prostate bed. Any legitimate prostate cancer treatment will destroy the cancer when it's confined to the gland. This last sentence bears repeating:

Any legitimate prostate cancer treatment will destroy cancer when it's confined to the gland.

All men should pay attention to the simple, low cost, painless tests that would virtually guarantee early detection, and therefore greatly increase chances for long-term disease-free survival.

Family History

In North America and in Western Europe, the chance of a man being diagnosed with prostate cancer is about 1 in 6. But, with a family history of the disease the risk increases dramatically.

In an article by Matthew Schmitz, M.D. (*About.com's Guide to Prostate Cancer*), male relatives of men with prostate cancer are at higher risk of developing prostate cancer. If your father had prostate cancer, your chance of developing the disease is 2.5 times greater than the norm. If your brother was affected, your chance is 3.2 times the norm. Also, according to Dr. Schmitz, ". . . the younger your relatives are when they develop prostate cancer, the greater your risk. If you have a first-degree relative who was diagnosed before the age of 65, then your risk increases over three times that of someone with no family history."

Others have simplified the family risk profile in the following table:

Normal Risk:	• One out of six (1/6)
With family history:	• 1 relative: risk doubles (2/6)
	• 2 relatives: five-fold increase (5/6)
	• 3 relatives: 97% chance (roughly 6/6)

Detecting Prostate Cancer

Following is a description of the way prostate cancer has been detected for the past 32 years, and, sadly, the same way it's being detected by most urologists today. Things are changing rapidly, however, and later chapters will address newer testing methods and techniques that are dramatically changing the way prostate cancer will be detected in the future. Many of these new techniques are available today, but unfortunately, few urologists have access to the tools and techniques.

The good news is, that armed with information presented in this book, any patient can take the appropriate steps to find a doctor or medical center that has invested in new testing equipment and is practicing new, state-of-the-art procedures for properly detecting prostate cancer.

Tip: Perhaps the strongest message in this book is that the patient should take control of his own health and cancer diagnosis. It's up to the patient to educate himself; arm himself with knowledge; ask the right questions; find the best doctor; and make a treatment decision that is in his best interest. For some, this may sound like an intimidating task, but it doesn't have to be. This book will guide you your journey. If you're uncomfortable doing this alone, enlist the help of a family member, friend or your primary care physician . . . anyone who may be able to assist you in taking control of your treatment decision. It's that important.

PSA Test

PSA refers to Prostate Specific Antigen. This is a protein secreted by the prostate gland, which "leaks" into the bloodstream. A simple blood test measures the level of this protein in nanograms per milliliter. The normal range for a healthy man is reported to be between 0 and 4.0. If you have a PSA reading of 1.5, it means there are 1.5 nanograms (that's 1.5 billionths of a gram) of the PSA protein, per milliliter (thousandth of a liter) in the blood sample.

PSA levels between 4 and 10 are generally considered "borderline." Levels above 10 are considered "high."

The conundrum here is that PSA is not an *absolute* indicator of prostate cancer. A borderline or even high PSA is no guarantee that cancer is present. Similarly, a PSA reading in the 0 to 4.0 range is no guarantee there's no cancer present.

However, studies have shown that this important test is often a *relative* indicator of the presence of cancer, and a caution flag should be raised if the number is beyond the normal range, or if a rapid rise is observed *even within the normal range.* You will learn later that PSA *velocity* – or the rate of increase – may be more important than the absolute value of your PSA.

PSA is also the key indicator of disease progression following treatment for prostate cancer.

Any stimulation of the prostate can cause PSA to temporarily rise producing a "red flag" and needless worry. Digital rectal exam and ejaculation stimulate the prostate and should be avoided for two to three days prior to the PSA blood test.

Tip: Avoid a digital rectal exam and sex for at least three days prior to having blood drawn for a PSA test to prevent an erroneous result.

Note: Before PSA testing was introduced, prostate cancer was not discovered in men until the disease was clinically advanced. And more than half the men diagnosed in those days had metastatic disease. The typical treatment for metastatic prostate cancer back then was bilateral orchiectomy. That's a fancy way of saying, "surgical removal of both testicles." Ouch!

Digital Rectal Exam

The digital rectal exam (DRE), a simple yet extremely important test is typically done by your internist during an annual physical exam. The doctor, wearing a rubber glove inserts his or her lubricated index finger into the anus and examines the prostate through the wall of the rectum.

A healthy prostate is generally small and supple. A diseased prostate can be enlarged with some indication of tumor presence. This can include abnormalities in texture, shape, or firmness. Often when a cancer has these characteristics, it has progressed beyond early stage.

Prostate cancer most frequently occurs near the periphery of the gland, so if a tumor is present, it can often be felt by DRE.

One limitation of this exam is that the finger can reach, and therefore examine, only the lateral and posterior (back) section of the prostate gland.

Most early stage prostate cancer patients have "normal feeling" prostates by DRE, and the cancer detection is done by means of a needle biopsy. Technology, however, is changing and detection techniques are improving dramatically. These new technologies will be discussed later in this book.

Transrectal Ultrasound

Another test used to determine abnormalities of the prostate is transrectal ultrasound (TRUS). In this examination, a small lubricated probe is inserted into the rectum. High frequency sound waves emitted from the probe bounce off the prostate gland creating echoes which are processed by computer and shown on a screen. Abnormalities not detectable by DRE can often be identified by TRUS. There's minimal discomfort and no pain associated with this simple and relatively quick test.

Biopsy

Typically, your internist would refer you to a urologist when either your PSA is elevated, or the DRE detects an abnormality. Your urologist would likely repeat the PSA blood test and the DRE. If either indicated the possibility of cancer, a biopsy would be ordered.

The prostate biopsy can be done one of three ways: transurethral (through the urethra), transrectal (through the rectum), or perineal (through the perineum, the space between the scrotum and the rectum). The transrectal biopsy is most common.

Transrectal Biopsy

A probe is inserted to provide an image of the prostate. This image is used to guide the probe to the exact spot desired to remove a tissue sample. A hollow needle passes through the wall of the rectum, into the prostate, and removes a core sample of tissue. This sample is packaged and labeled as to its location within the gland. Using this same technique, several more samples are taken from both lobes of the prostate and then sent to a pathology laboratory for examination.

If cancer is present, the pathology report will identify the specific type of cancer and the estimated percentage of the sample involved. The lab will also grade the cancer according to its level of aggressiveness. The grading system is referred to as the Gleason score. Lower Gleason scores generally indicate early stage, non-aggressive cancers. Higher Gleason scores point to more potent malignancies.

Depending on several factors, a doctor may order additional tests to determine if the cancer has metastasized (spread beyond the prostate bed). For example, in the case of a borderline or high PSA, the presence of a palpable tumor by DRE and/or a moderate-to-high Gleason score, the doctor would likely order a bone scan, CT scan, or PET scan to look for the disease in other parts of the body.

Although not especially painful, the transrectal ultrasound-guided needle biopsy is not an enjoyable experience. There can be some rectal discomfort for a few hours following the procedure, along with the presence of blood in the urine, stool, or ejaculate for several days to a few weeks.

Bone Scan

The bone scan is a 2-dimensional image of the skeleton using a radioactive tracer. This is a common test to detect cancer that has spread to the bone, a favorite site for prostate cancer to go.

A scan of your skeleton helps determine if cancer has spread to the pelvis, lower spine, or other bone structures in the body.

CT Scan

Computerized tomography (CT) is a 3-dimensional image of the body using X-rays. CT is a commonly used tool to help detect cancer that has metastasized beyond the tissue or organ from where it started. CT is useful when looking for the spread of cancer into the nearby bone and lymph nodes.

PET Scan

Positron emission tomography (PET) scans are performed to identify the presence of tumors. Radioactive glucose or other compounds are injected and tend to concentrate in tumor locations.

Chest X-Ray

Chest X-ray (CXR) is a 2-dimensional image of the lung, ribs, and back bone using x-rays. A CXR is commonly used to detect the spread of cancer to the chest area and for screening for other diseases.

MRI

Magnetic Resonance Imaging (MRI) is a 3-dimensional image of the body using magnets and radio waves that is very different from a CT. Some of our tissues and organs are seen better by a CT, some by MRI and some by combining both. MRI is useful to detect the spread of cancer in the soft tissues.

Advances in These Technologies

As mentioned above, there have been significant advances in some of these technologies since the first edition of this book and will be discussed in later chapters. To call these advances "game changers" is an understatement.

Early Detection Summary

One of the most important messages in this book is that *early detection* greatly improves your chance of a cure. I cannot over emphasize the importance of early detection. If the cancer is identified before it spreads outside the gland the chances of a complete cure are virtually guaranteed. Also, by catching the cancer early, you have *all* the treatment options available to you. If, on the other hand, your cancer has spread to the margins, the seminal vesicles or the lymph nodes, treatment becomes increasingly more difficult, your options become more limited, and chances of a durable and complete remission are diminished.

Tip: The most important thing a man can do to ensure early detection is to have annual physical examinations that include blood PSA measurement and DRE.

Other symptoms in the prostate region, such as urination difficulty, burning during urination, or pain in the pelvic region, should be called to the immediate attention of your internist or urologist.

Treatment Options

Once you've been diagnosed with prostate cancer the world doesn't come to an end. *Prostate cancer is not a death sentence.* In fact, prostate cancer is not like many other cancers. Caught early it can be cured with a high degree of certainty. Even when diagnosed in mid and later stages it can often be effectively treated and cured.

Most newly diagnosed men I communicate with are fortunate enough to have been diagnosed with early stage disease. Nevertheless, they're typically frightened and confused. I often try to lighten things up by telling them: "If you're going to have cancer, prostate cancer is the one to have. And, if you're going to have prostate cancer, the numbers don't get much better than yours." This usually is the case, and it puts men – and their wives – at ease and makes it much easier to begin exploring treatment options with them.

When prostate cancer has been diagnosed, you have many options available:

1. *Radical Prostatectomy*, or the surgical removal of the prostate. There are two types of radical prostatectomy:
   - Open surgery
   - Laparoscopic surgery

2. *External Beam Radiation Therapy,* or *EBRT.* There are several forms of radiation therapy including:

   - Conventional External Beam Radiation Therapy
   - Conformal External Beam Radiation Therapy
   - IMRT (Intensity Modulated Radiation Therapy)
   - IGRT (Image Guided Radiation Therapy)
   - SBRT (Stereotactic Body Radiation Therapy). The most common form of SBRT is CyberKnife
   - RapidArc
   - Tomotherapy
   - Proton Therapy
   - Others

3. *Internal Radiation Therapy,* called *Brachytherapy,* which refers to radioactive seed implants. There are two types of Brachytherapy.
   - *Permanent seed implants*
   - *Removable seeds,* called *HDR Brachytherapy*

4. *Cryosurgery* – Liquid nitrogen freezing of the cancer

5. *HIFU* - High Intensity Focused Ultrasound

6. *Hormone Ablation Therapy (or Androgen Deprivation Therapy)* – The use of one or more hormones to shut down the production of male hormones, such as testosterone, that feed the cancer

7. *Chemotherapy.* The use of anti-cancer drugs to slow or stop the growth of rapidly dividing cancer cells in the body.

8. *Immunotherapy.* This refers to harnessing the power of your body's natural defenses to fight cancer cells.

9. *Active Surveillance* (sometimes called *Watchful Waiting*). This is technically not a "treatment," but it's a perfectly acceptable course of action for early stage cancer as we will discuss later.

Chemotherapy and immunotherapy are typically used for advanced or recurrent cancers and will not be discussed in detail here. The other common treatment options will be discussed in detail in later chapters.

How Do You Know if You're Cured?

Once you have chosen one of the above treatments, how do you know if it worked? There is disagreement in the medical community on this subject. Cancer is much different from other medical conditions. When a broken bone is repaired, you know it. When heart bypass surgery is completed you know the restriction has been eliminated. When an infection has been destroyed, analytical measurements can confirm this.

But cancer is insidious, in that microscopic cells can linger close to the original cancer site or can migrate through different channels to other parts of the body. There they can establish colonies and continue their dirty work. For that reason, cancer patients need to be monitored for some time to determine if the cancer has been completely removed or destroyed.

For prostate cancer patients, the best measure is PSA. PSA in the blood can come from only two places – prostate tissue or prostate cancer cells. In the case of surgery, where the prostate is removed, a patient's PSA should drop to zero – or less than 0.1 ng/mL, the detectable limit. A result higher than that is an indication of prostate cancer – or laboratory error. The latter possibility is always a reason to repeat the blood test and lab analysis.

When the prostate is left in place, as is the case for all other treatment options, there will usually be some PSA in the blood from a functioning, or even partially functioning prostate gland. But increasing levels of PSA are of concern. For this reason, PSA is still the primary measure of cancer activity, backed up with periodic digital rectal exams (DREs) – but PSA is treated differently in this case.

All forms of radiation, as well as cryosurgery, damage cancer cell DNA. Damaged DNA results in something called apoptosis, or programmed cell death, or in necrosis, another form of cell death. The damaged cancer cells will live for some time, but they cannot reproduce and therefore eventually die off.

For these patients, PSA is tracked periodically, usually every six months, for several years.

There are two terms used by physicians to report on success or failure of prostate cancer treatment: bNED and cNED.

bNED, refers to no *biochemical* evidence of disease. The American Society for Therapeutic Radiology and Oncology (ASTRO) considers one to be biochemically free of prostate cancer as long as the patient's PSA remains essentially flat after it reaches its low point, or nadir. If PSA rises by more than 2 ng/mL over the nadir, one *may* have experienced *biochemical* failure, i.e., prostate cancer may have returned. This is referred to as the *Phoenix* definition of biochemical failure.

The term cNED refers to no *clinical* evidence of disease. The clinical test for disease is the digital rectal exam (DRE). If the physician notices a lump by DRE, in a patient where there was no prior lump; or if an existing lump (tumor) is growing larger, the patient may have experienced *clinical* failure. Before the PSA test was available, the DRE was the only test available to monitor progress following treatment for prostate cancer.

bNED and cNED are used in combination to monitor cure rates for prostate cancer patients. Generally speaking, the lower the nadir post treatment, the better are the chances of long term bNED and cNED (i.e., cure). Studies of radiation-treated patients typically

18

compare patients with nadirs in three categories: 1) PSA less than 0.5, 2) 0.5 to 1.0 and, 3) greater than 1.0. The first category, less than 0.5 post treatment, is clearly the most desirable.

Become Your Own Advocate

As stated earlier, this is perhaps the most important message in this book. *You need to take charge of your own treatment decision.* No single treatment is best for everybody. In the case of prostate cancer, you have several treatment alternatives, and there is only one person on this planet who is qualified to choose the option that is best for you – *You!* But you need to do your homework first, so you are comfortable with your decision.

Most of us were brought up to believe the doctor knows best. One of the most common questions a prostate cancer patient asks his doctor is "What would you do if you were me, doctor?" And the doctor will tell you. But what you need to realize is that doctors in different specialties will often give you different answers to that question. Let me repeat this very important point:

Tip: Doctors in different specialties will often give you different answers to the question, "What would you do doc?" And most are biased to their specialty.

In the course of my interviews of hundreds of prostate cancer patients, the vast majority reported that when they met with their urologist, who is fundamentally a surgeon, surgery was recommended. The radiation oncologist typically recommended radiation. Those who met with doctors specializing in brachytherapy were generally encouraged to do seed implants. Cryo-surgeons recommended freezing, and so on. How can surgery, external beam radiation, seeds and liquid nitrogen all be *best* for the same patient? They can't.

Does this mean that doctors are intentionally misleading their patients for their own personal gain? No. Most doctors will act in terms of what they believe is in the best interest of their patients. Sadly, many doctors are not knowledgeable about some of the developing technologies. Therefore, it is up to you, the patient, to do your own homework, and make the treatment decision that is best for *you*.

I chose proton beam therapy (PBT, a form of external beam radiation) for my treatment. My urologist, who is chief of urology for a major hospital in the Northeast, admitted lack of knowledge of proton beam treatment and encouraged me to have surgery. Why? Because he was very experienced; he had performed several hundred radical prostatectomies; and he believed that, considering my age, physical condition, PSA, and Gleason score, surgery offered me the best chance for a cure.

The radiation oncologist, said, "Considering your age, cancer stage, and general health, I recommend conformal external beam radiation therapy."

The brachytherapist felt similarly about his specialty. He told me that I was "the poster boy for brachytherapy." Why? Because of my relatively young age, good health, non-enlarged prostate, early stage cancer, and his experience and expertise at his specialty.

The doctor I spoke with about cryosurgery felt the same way. If he were in my shoes, he would choose to freeze the prostate.

How could each of these treatment options be best for me? I knew they couldn't. They might all have worked, but what about such issues as impotence, incontinence, fatigue, pain, convenience, cost, treatment time, recuperation time, and other factors that were important to me?

I quickly learned one of the most important lessons of this journey: *The only way I can know for sure what's best for me is to jump in with both feet, learn everything I can about each option and then make my own decision.* I did this, and my ultimate decision surprised everyone – especially me.

When I was first diagnosed with prostate cancer and did my preliminary research, proton beam therapy (PBT) wasn't even on my radar screen. I didn't know it existed. I now lead a 10,000-member international support group for men who have chosen PBT. I therefore admit a built-in bias toward this option. But I do not think it is for everybody. And I truly believe that by reading and understanding what is presented in this book, you too will make the decision that is best for you.

Commonly Asked Questions

There are two questions men and their partners often think about and are afraid or embarrassed to ask. The first: "Is there any connection between the level of a man's sexual activity (i.e. the *use* of the prostate) and prostate cancer?" The answer is – maybe. The fact is, both sexually active men and celibate men develop prostate cancer. But, in recent years there is a growing body of evidence that frequent sex (ejaculation) may help prevent prostate cancer.

A Harvard University study involving 29,342 men ages 46 to 81 concluded that, "men who ejaculated 21 or more times a month enjoyed a 33 percent lower risk of prostate cancer compared with men who reported four to seven ejaculations a month throughout their lifetimes."

The second question: "If I am diagnosed with prostate cancer, can I give it to my wife or partner when we have sex?" The answer is no. Prostate cancer is not contagious or transmittable during intercourse.

Summary

You must take charge of your own case in order to make the best decision for *you*. Prostate cancer is different from other cancers, and prostate cancer treatment options are all very different from each other.

In the case of prostate cancer, *you* need to take control of the decision-making process. Doing so can make a world of difference in the success of your treatment and in the quality of your life following treatment. The remainder of this book is about what you need to do to take control of the detection and treatment of prostate cancer.

CHAPTER 2

My Early Indications of Prostate Cancer

*"The beginning of knowledge is the discovery
of something we do not understand."*

– Frank Herbert

Dad Was First

I was a little boy when my father had his operation. Back then you didn't say the word "cancer" in our house. The word wasn't allowed in our vocabulary. Occasionally my mother would refer to the dreaded disease as "The Big C."

My father's operation for prostate cancer was kept a secret from friends and family. Not even his four children were told why he was in the hospital. He was just having surgery on his "private parts."

He survived the operation and, over time, had no indications of cancer recurrence. Of course, this was before PSA was measured, so we didn't know for sure if the cancer was still growing in his body. Years later, he also survived colon cancer – another secret that was kept from the children. And when he passed away in 1979, it was from a stroke – totally unrelated to his two encounters with "The Big C." I later learned how important a role heredity plays in the cancer puzzle, and how much more vigilant my brother and I should have been.

The Early Signs Were There

Physical fitness was always important to me. I always paid attention to my diet and began jogging for health in my early 30s. From that time forward, I ran and exercised 4 to 6 days a week.

Annual physicals were also a part of my regimen beginning at age 40. Before then my physicals were randomly spaced.

I monitored my blood pressure, cholesterol level, triglycerides and other factors. It wasn't until my early 50s that I started paying attention to my PSA.

Not much had been published about PSA in the 1970s and 80s. But its validity as a prostate cancer marker was becoming more and more accepted.

As far back as I can recall, my PSA was on the high side of "normal." The early measurements ranged from about 2.5 to 3.5. Nothing to be alarmed about – or so I was told. I didn't know then that I was at high risk, and perhaps should have been biopsied years earlier because of my family history.

In my mid-50s, my PSA began to rise a little faster, approaching 4.0.

My Brother's Turn

Coincidentally, my older brother by six years, Gene, had been experiencing rising PSA. Routine DREs did not detect any abnormalities in his prostate. However, when his PSA moved beyond the normal range, his urologist ordered a needle biopsy. The results came back positive for prostate cancer.

Gene then did what most of us would do. He consulted his urologist. "Go with the 'gold standard,' surgery," the doctor advised. Gene, a busy businessman, took that advice and his radical prostatectomy was set for one month later. This gave him time to "bank" four pints of blood in the event he needed it during surgery. As it turned out, he needed six pints.

His wife, Toni, and I were with him just before surgery and I remember the worried look on his face. Gene, being justifiably frightened, always a bit melodramatic – and now in the role of the family patriarch – began lecturing me on my responsibilities. "If

24

anything happens to me, Bob, you need to step into my role. Make sure mom is taken care of, help Toni handle my affairs; keep an eye on my kids; and stay close to your sisters." Until then, I hadn't given much thought to my brother's, or my own mortality. It was a sobering experience. I wasn't ready for – and I didn't want – the patriarch role.

They wheeled Gene in for surgery while Toni and I waited. I knew enough about the procedure to understand this was *major* surgery, and there were always chances of complications. So, we stayed at the hospital to await the outcome.

Four hours later it was over, and Gene was brought into the recovery room. A short time later, Toni and I were allowed to visit him. We were told the operation went well, and that he was still groggy from the anesthesia. In retrospect, that visit had a monumental impact on me.

At first, I didn't recognize my brother. He seemed to have shriveled in size. The tubes and wires attached to him were intimidating. It was hard to believe this was my big brother, the guy who always beat me at every game we played; the patriarch; the cornerstone of our family.

Tip: If you've decided on surgery as treatment for your prostate cancer, do not visit a friend or relative who has recently had a radical prostatectomy. A visit to a patient soon after his surgery may change your mind.

Tip: If you're looking for a reason to eliminate surgery as an option, visit someone who has had this procedure soon after his operation.

I Could Be Next

It was then I realized I might be in for a similar fate, because my PSA was rising.

While in the recovery room with my brother, I decided that if I were ever diagnosed with prostate cancer, I'd make every effort to find an alternative to surgery to avoid the trauma, blood loss, and side effects.

Radical prostatectomy just seemed too barbaric to me. Even the term "radical" instills fear. The prostate is located deep inside the torso; lots of "parts" need to be displaced to access this gland; it's surrounded by delicate organs that are critical to maintaining sexual function and bladder control; and the operation can be extremely bloody.

PSA Rising

My PSA continued to rise, and when it broke through the "magic" 4.0 and hit 4.2, my internist recommended I see a urologist.

The urologist performed a DRE, which was normal. He next did an ultrasound, which indicated a normal-sized prostate with no unusual characteristics. And finally, he took a blood sample for PSA. The lab results confirmed the initial 4.2 reading. The urologist told me he wasn't particularly concerned but suggested I retest my PSA in six months.

I later learned that I was at high risk, and that a biopsy should have been ordered at that time, or even a year earlier, when my PSA had risen from 3.1 to 3.9 – a red flag.

The six-month PSA was 4.6. It was time for a needle biopsy.

My First Biopsy

This was an interesting experience, to say the least. First of all, I didn't know there were different techniques involved in taking biopsy samples. Neither did I know that the number of biopsy samples taken varied from urologist to urologist, from as few as 6 samples to as many as 24. Nor did I know that I could have opted for local anesthesia to ease the pain and discomfort.

My urologist told me the biopsy would be quick and relatively painless; and though it might be a little uncomfortable, it would be over before I knew it. As it turned out, he was wrong on all counts. He informed me he was planning to insert an ultrasound tube in my rectum to produce an image of my prostate to help determine where to take samples. While the tube was inserted, he said he would insert another device, a spring-loaded hollow needle, which would pass through my rectal wall, into my prostate and remove samples for analysis.

I remember saying, "You mean to tell me that you're going to fire a dart through my rectum, and rip out a chunk of my prostate?" He said, "Well that's one way to put it." "How many times will you do this?" I wanted to know. "Six," he replied. "Are you sure it won't hurt?" I asked. "Well, it might hurt a little. But it'll be over before you know it." Wrong and wrong. It later occurred to me that he would have no way of knowing if it hurt or not. He had never been on the receiving end of this procedure!

The morning of the biopsy, I didn't have much of an appetite for breakfast. I had some juice and coffee, took the antibiotic prescribed to prevent infection, and drove to the urologist's office.

As directed, I removed my clothes, climbed up on the table and rolled over on my left side. I was feeling particularly vulnerable, knowing, I thought, what would happen next.

This urologist worked alone, which I later discovered was a big disadvantage for me. He began by inserting a large diameter tube that felt like an aluminum baseball bat. Next, came his vintage ultrasound probe. Then he inserted the spring-loaded needle. It felt as though everything on his shelf was being loaded into my rectal cavity. Next, he fired the first shot. Snap! That's the sound you hear while you experience a strange sensation in your lower rectum, similar to an instantaneous, somewhat painful hemorrhoid.

Things got worse. Because he worked alone, he had no one to package and label the sample. So, he had to remove the needle, the ultrasound probe, the baseball bat, and the other paraphernalia.

After packaging and labeling the sample, he re-inserted the entire ensemble and repeated the procedure – *five more times*. This less-than-pleasant procedure took about 30 minutes. What ever happened to, "It'll be over before you know it?"

Tip: Before having a prostate biopsy, find out if your doctor does this procedure alone, or if he has an assistant. If he works alone, find another urologist. This procedure can be completed in less than ten minutes with two people working together – one sampling, the other packaging and labeling.

I can't say that the procedure was *extremely* painful. Some men claim it's "a piece of cake" (remind me to avoid their bakery). But for me, and others I have interviewed, it was uncomfortable at the very least. Some say it was very uncomfortable, and even painful.

One study from the Urological Institute at the Cleveland Clinic reported that up to 96 percent of patients who undergo prostate biopsy report pain.

After the procedure, I was left with what can best be described as a "bad headache" in my rectum. After an over-the-counter pain killer and a few hours of rest the pain was gone, but not the side effects. For about two weeks I had blood in my urine, ejaculate and stool. This is not unusual following a prostate biopsy.

Tip: Some urologists use a local anesthetic to eliminate pain during prostate biopsy. Find a urologist who will do this. It will make all the difference in the world in your comfort level during this procedure.

My theory on this subject is the following: A urologist with a helper can typically perform about four biopsies per hour. That is, if no anesthetic is used. Using a local anesthetic, such as topical lidocaine gel or a periprostatic injectable anesthetic, to minimize or eliminate pain, slows things down because the doctor must wait for the patient to "numb up." So, the urologist can perform only about two prostate biopsies per hour, thus, his reluctance to recommend a local anesthetic. After all, it doesn't hurt the urologist one bit.

Bottom line: the better educated the patient, the more comfortable the patient and the fewer surprises.

First Biopsy Results

This next part was difficult. My heart goes out to anyone who has ever had a biopsy – prostate or otherwise – the waiting is *torture*. A week went by and I called the doctor's office as requested. I braced myself for the worst and prayed for the best.

The doctor was not in, but his office manager told me she would look up the results. Her search took about three minutes, which felt like three hours. "Good news," she said. "The biopsy was negative."

I gasped as I let out the breath I had been inadvertently holding, and I thanked her profusely – as if she had something to do with the wonderful results.

Later, the doctor called me and told me he wanted to see me again in a year.

My PSA Continues to Rise

A year later my PSA had risen to 5.2 and my urologist ordered another biopsy.

By this time, I had done a little research. I had learned that other urologists worked with biopsy sampling specialists using more modern and, thankfully, smaller equipment, and more streamlined techniques.

I decided to switch urologists and chose one who was a prominent physician in a well-known Boston hospital. His technique was no "walk in the park," but it was infinitely better than my previous doctor's procedure.

With coffee, juice and antibiotic in place, I drove to the urologist's office, and for some reason, I was less apprehensive than the first time I went through this routine.

I didn't have to remove my clothes; I just climbed up on the table, slid my pants and shorts below my knees; and rolled over onto my left side. A much smaller broomstick-sized device was inserted in my now highly explored rectum. The ultrasound probe and spring-loaded needle were inserted in tandem.

A sample was taken. Snap. Then another. Snap. And then four more Snap. Snap. Snap, Snap. The two men talked and joked during the procedure, which actually relaxed me. I found myself joining in the conversation and joking along with them. Five or six minutes later it was over. Having a two-man team permitted them to grab and package the samples without having to remove and reinsert the "broomstick," which made the entire ordeal much more tolerable and of significantly shorter duration. This pleased me to no end – pun intended. Yes, there was some pain, but less than before, and it was over so quickly, I didn't really have time to think about it.

Tip: Talk with others who have been biopsied. Find out if their doctors used the most modern equipment and procedure. Determine how long the procedure took and how much discomfort they experienced. A prostate biopsy doesn't have to be painful.

Despite the dramatically improved equipment and procedure, the side effects were the same. Soreness for several hours, plus blood in my urine, stool and ejaculate.

Second Biopsy Results

Another week of torture. This time I knew I'd get the news while cruising the Atlantic with two friends. We were running a boat up to Massachusetts from South Florida. During the trip, I was a bit preoccupied with the news I'd be receiving that week. I had a gnawing feeling the test results would be positive and I'd be told I had prostate cancer. I kept picturing my brother in the recovery room. Then I saw myself in his place with tubes, drains, catheters and such. *Not a pretty picture.*

We were off the coast of North Carolina when I called my doctor's office from the cell phone on the designated day. The receptionist put me in touch with a nurse who told me she couldn't lay her hands on my test results and suggested I call back in an hour. . . *60 more agonizing minutes.*

I called back. This time she had the results, and again, good news – the biopsy was negative! I remember telling this woman that I loved her, and I would be sending her flowers.

We had dinner that night on the boat, and I recall having an extra martini with my friends to celebrate the good news.

But I still had to face one indisputable fact. My PSA was rising, and that wasn't good.

CHAPTER 3

The Dreaded Diagnosis

"You must live in the world as it is."
– Dean Acheson

PSA Rises Further – and Now a *Free* PSA Signal

Six months later my PSA was 6.6 and six months after that, it had reached 7.5. To add to my fears, my doctor ordered a relatively new test called *Free* PSA. This is a test that measures the amount of unbound, or "free" prostate-specific antigen in the blood. It helps determine the degree to which high PSA may be related to cancer versus other benign conditions.

In my case, both numbers were where they shouldn't be. PSA was now 7.9, and free PSA was low at 7 percent, indicating a 56 percent probability that I had prostate cancer.

It was time for another biopsy.

This time I went to the same urologist and he used the same technique – uncomfortable, but tolerable. And I had the same side effects.

Tip: If you have rapidly rising PSA, whether or not it's outside the normal range and whether or not you have an abnormal DRE, have your doctor instruct the laboratory to run a "free PSA" test in addition to the standard PSA test. It costs a few dollars more, but it can provide valuable data indicating the probability of prostate cancer, well before a biopsy is called for. Newer, and more precise tests will be discussed later.

Third Biopsy Results – 'The Big C'

It was August 2000. I was with my wife and a group of friends vacationing in Nantucket on my boat. Since I was expecting bad news this time, I told my doctor I would call him for the test results *after* I returned from vacation a week later – I really didn't want to know the results until I returned home.

Unfortunately, my doctor forgot my request. On Thursday, August 10, 2000, I decided to check my messages at home using my cell phone. There were five messages, one of which I remember clearly: "Mr. Marckini, this is 'Dr. Parker.' I have your biopsy results and I'd like you and your wife to meet with me in my office this Friday. Please call for an appointment." Not the most sensitive way to deliver an obvious and ominous message.

This message could mean only one thing. I have "The Big C." My heart pounded; my mouth went dry; and all the color went out of my world. Suddenly, everything was moving in slow motion. My wife was with me when I retrieved my messages and she instantly knew what had happened from the expression on my face. "I have prostate cancer, honey," I said.

I told her I wasn't going to call the doctor and spoil the rest of our vacation. I just didn't want to hear those words from him, even though I knew what he was going to say. But my wife persuaded me to make the call. "Why torture yourself and me? You've got to make that call." I tried to come up with an argument to support my position, but I knew she was right.

So, I called and here is what I heard: "Mr. Marckini, your biopsy results came back, and you have prostate cancer. Two of the eight samples tested positively for adenocarcinoma. The good news is that we caught it at an early stage. Less than 5 percent of your prostate is involved."

The rest of the conversation was a blur. After he told me I had cancer I didn't really hear anything else he said.

We set up an appointment for the following week so we could finish our vacation in Nantucket. But the vacation really ended with that phone call. We stayed a few more days, but my mind was on cancer, surgery, blood loss, impotence, incontinence . . . and death.

Communicating with Family and Friends

I remember telling two of our closest friends and fighting back tears as I gave them the details. This wasn't going to be easy. I was frightened and it showed. My wife asked me if it would be easier for me if she told our other friends who were vacationing with us. Sheepishly, I said yes. It was awkward for a couple of days. But by the time vacation was over, we were discussing my prostate cancer with our friends, casually over dinner.

Frequently, in the back of my mind, however, I could see the haunting image of my brother in the recovery room, and I pictured myself in his place. It was a nightmare.

Telling my two daughters I had prostate cancer was one of the most difficult things I've ever had to do. This was complicated by the fact that we were planning my younger daughter's wedding, only a few weeks away.

"Oh, my God," I thought, "Will I be able to walk her down the aisle?" It's amazing the things that go through your head when you get news like this.

I waited until vacation was over, when I could tell them face-to-face. I also wanted more time to get used to the idea, so I would sound matter of fact about it, and not worry them. After all, I kept telling myself, it *was* early stage cancer and I was only 57 years old and in excellent health.

My daughters handled the news well and committed their prayers and support, which was exactly what I needed. I received similar responses from my friends and relatives.

It Was There All the Time

I later learned that cancer takes years to grow, and that it was certainly present in my prostate two years before, when I had my first biopsy. Then why didn't the doctor find it? Because he took only six samples, three in each lobe. Certainly, if he had taken more samples, the chances of finding the cancer would have been much greater.

Some doctors, I discovered, routinely take eight samples; others take 12; and some more progressive urologists remove 24 tissue samples. If you think about it, the chances of finding microscopic cancer cells increases manyfold with a larger number of samples.

Look at it this way: Picture a football stadium filled five feet deep with several billion white marbles – which represent normal, healthy cells. Now, from a plane, sprinkle a few hundred black marbles (representing cancer cells) over the stadium and mix them in with a bulldozer. Next, picture yourself going into the stadium blindfolded and carrying a shovel. What are your chances of finding some black marbles if you remove only six shovels-full of marbles? Pretty slim. Certainly, the more samples you take, the greater your chances of finding some of the black marbles. The same is true when doing a prostate biopsy.

Rising PSA tells you there *may* be cancer cells in your prostate. In early stage prostate cancer, there's typically no detectable tumor or lump on which to focus the biopsy needle. This is much different from other forms of cancer, such as breast cancer, where a lump or lesion is usually evident. With breast cancer, the biopsy needle can be directed to the suspicious area.

If there is cancer in your prostate, it's to your *great* advantage to find it early. Early cancer detection means a) more treatment options, b) better chance of a cure, and c) better quality of life after treatment.

A recent study published in the *Daily University Science News* pointed out that one in seven cancers is missed by traditional biopsy sampling (I suspect it's worse than one in seven) – all the more reason for increasing the number of samples taken.

If cancer is present, your PSA will continue to rise, and you will be facing the unpleasant biopsy experience again. So why put yourself through the trauma of multiple biopsies needlessly? If the cancer is there, you want to find it – and you want to find it early.

There's one more reason for taking a larger number of biopsy samples. If the pathology results do, in fact, come back negative, you are much more confident that there really is no cancer present, and you can rest easy.

Tip: If you're going to have a prostate biopsy, insist on a minimum of 12 samples. And insist on local anesthesia to prevent pain and discomfort. More on this subject later.

Note: In later chapters we'll discuss new, state-of-the-art imaging techniques that are giving doctors a *much* clearer picture of cancer activity and location. Perhaps it won't be necessary to take as many samples as these imaging tests improve.

Looking back, and knowing what I know now, here are some facts that would have altered my thinking and my approach to diagnosis:

1. My father had prostate cancer. This *doubled* my chance of being diagnosed.

2. My older brother was diagnosed with prostate cancer. With two close relatives having been diagnosed, my chances were *five times greater* than the average man.

3. The rapid rise in my PSA (more than 0.75 ng/mL in one year) was one more indicator that cancer was present more than two years before it was diagnosed.

4. When my brother was diagnosed, my PSA was in the high end of the normal range. Considering all the other factors, the probability I had prostate cancer was quite high.

If I knew then what I know now, I have zero doubt that my cancer would have been detected years earlier.

Why is this important? Simply because the earlier you diagnose this disease, the higher the probability the cancer is still localized and curable. I was fortunate that mine was *still* discovered relatively early. However, if my doctor – or I – had been more alert, or better informed, I would have been diagnosed at a time that would have substantially improved my chance of a long-term cure.

Tip: You should become your own advocate when it comes to protecting yourself from this disease. You should learn what you need to know about what puts you at higher risk for prostate cancer. You should take responsibility for tracking your own PSA. And, you should have a competent physician working with you in this process. The information presented in this book will teach you how to do all these things.

CHAPTER 4

My Preliminary Research

"Out of your vulnerabilities will come your strength."
– Sigmund Freud

As an engineer, I was accustomed to collecting data, dealing with technical information, evaluating pros and cons of options, and making decisions. My problem, however, was not a lack of information; it was the opposite – an overwhelming *abundance* of information. And most disconcerting, in my early research, was the fact that no option seemed to emerge as the preferred choice. They all had significant drawbacks.

Between the time I received the phone call with the diagnosis, and my first meeting with the urologist, I devoured everything I could find on prostate cancer treatment. I wanted to be prepared for the meeting with all the information I could gather, including a list of all the important questions.

I began by making calls to all the people I knew who had dealt with this dreaded disease. Each one of them gave me the name of two or three people they knew who were treated for prostate cancer. The list grew and grew, and there was one common theme. All these men had chosen surgery – radical prostatectomy. Was it going to be as simple as this?

But what about the promise I made myself that day in the recovery room, standing beside my brother following his surgery?

Tip: When doing your own research, make sure you talk with several men who have been treated by each of the major treatment options – not just surgery. I can't overemphasize how important this is in your own personal treatment decision. Spend

time with them. Take them out to lunch. Much useful information comes out after the first few minutes of polite conversation.

With the exception of one of these men, they all informed me of the seriousness of the surgery, the discomfort they experienced following their treatment, and the lingering side effects they were dealing with. The most common side effect reported was partial to complete loss of sexual function, followed closely by varying degrees of incontinence, or loss of bladder control. One individual – a healthy, athletic 63-year-old – told me the operation was "no big deal," that he experienced no side effects, and that he felt he had made the right decision. My research continued.

While I made telephone calls, I continued to work the Internet. I discovered that surgery was the most common treatment recommended by urologists, followed by various forms of radiation including external beam (X-ray) radiation and brachytherapy (radioactive seed implantation). There was also reference to cryoablation using liquid nitrogen to kill the cancer by freezing it.

Another approach chosen by some men is essentially doing nothing, except monitoring the situation. This is called "watchful waiting," or "active surveillance." Under certain circumstances, I learned, this can be a reasonable approach.

Somewhere in the thousands of pages of Internet literature there was a passing reference to a treatment called proton beam therapy. The information was limited in scope and offered minimal details. At the time, I assumed proton therapy was experimental and investigational. Nevertheless, I downloaded and printed what I found, and put it aside in my office.

Help from The Caribbean – A Major Turning Point

Early in this process I received a call from a good friend, who was retired and living on his sailboat in the Caribbean. Larry had recently been diagnosed with prostate cancer and had chosen surgery on his urologist's recommendation. He also suffered some of the typical side effects. I had emailed Larry notifying him of my diagnosis. He received my message on his wireless computer system

38

somewhere off the coast of Grenada. A couple of days later he called me.

Larry reinforced my resolve to try to find an alternative to surgery as he related details of his lingering side effects. In the same conversation he told me the story of his friend Max, a Caribbean boating acquaintance who had recently been treated for prostate cancer. I didn't realize it at the time, but this conversation turned out to be a major turning point in my search for the best treatment.

Proton Treatment Is Real

Larry told me that he and Max had been treated for prostate cancer at about the same time. Weeks later, when both were in the Caribbean, Larry was out for his daily walk, still tender from his surgery, when Max jogged by. Larry was dumbfounded, as he had assumed Max had also chosen surgery.

When Larry inquired, he learned that Max had chosen proton therapy, and this treatment involved no pain, no blood loss, no trauma and no discomfort. Max, in fact, told Larry he jogged each day *while he was in treatment.*

When Larry heard this, he couldn't wait to tell me about his discovery. He knew I was doing research and needed to make a treatment decision. He also knew I was searching for an alternative to surgery.

I told Larry I had heard about proton treatment, but I hadn't really gotten into it in much detail. He told me that although this procedure was relatively new, he heard it was not experimental; the cure rates were comparable to surgery; and it was covered by medical insurance. Most exciting to me was the fact that Max reported experiencing *no side effects whatsoever.*

During the phone conversation with Larry, I dug through my research material and found the scant, few pages on proton therapy I had downloaded from the Internet. The information was interesting, but after reading it I still had more questions than answers.

I asked Larry for Max's cell phone number and called him. We spent about 45 minutes on the phone, and he answered all my questions. Max was a well-educated, successful, retired businessman, and as such, his decision to choose protons gave this option much credence. He had done his homework.

39

His urologist had recommended surgery, but Max put that on hold while he evaluated other options. He read everything he could on the subject, and he visited Loma Linda University Cancer Center (LLUCC) in Southern California to meet with the doctors and staff.

Max recounted the details of his treatment and told me about his life-changing experience with proton therapy.

When I finished talking with Max, I was excited – "Maybe this is it," I thought. But being a "recovering engineer," I knew I had a lot more work to do.

In the meantime, I had to meet with my urologist for the first time since my positive biopsy. I knew from my brother's experience that the doctor would recommend surgery. I wanted to ask the right questions, so I did a quick study of this procedure called radical prostatectomy.

Meeting with My Urologist

The day came, and my wife and I met with my urologist – one of the finest in his profession in the northeast. He pointed out that I was fortunate – my cancer was early stage. He told me that my tumor stage was T1c and my Gleason score was "only a 3+2, or 5." The way he said this sounded like I should feel good about it. I was just beginning to learn about Gleason score and realized this was in the middle of the range, but I didn't know much more than that.

Next, he told me that my physical health and relative youth (57 years old!) made me an ideal candidate for surgery, with an excellent chance of full recovery. He even used a term I would hear several more times during my due diligence. He told me I was the "poster boy" for radical prostatectomy (RP).

When I asked about alternatives to surgery, he indicated there were a few, but I should seriously consider only two – brachytherapy (seeds) or external beam radiation therapy (EBRT). He gave me the name of physicians in these specialties and suggested I speak with them.

"If I choose surgery, when could you do it?" I asked. "No sooner than four weeks from now, as you need to bank four units of your own blood," he replied. Immediately, I pictured my weakened brother in the recovery room after losing six pints of blood.

I thought it was time to ask him the question that was burning in my mind. "Doctor, I've been doing some research and I came across something called proton therapy, and it looks quite interesting."

His reaction caught me totally off guard. He brushed it off and said, "That's experimental. You could damage your rectum and wind up needing a colostomy."

I was devastated. A colostomy, I knew, was a surgical procedure where a section of the colon is brought out through an opening in the abdomen. Stools pass into a small bag fastened over the opening.

I felt like I had been kicked in the stomach. That statement certainly deflated my enthusiasm for the treatment that seemed so right for me. But I pressed on, asking more questions about proton therapy. I told him about what I had read, and what I had heard from a former patient. He changed the subject and told us to go home and think about the three "legitimate" options we had discussed. We left with some documents to read and forms to sign.

Driving home, I began to think that what I'd been reading about proton therapy was all hype. Maybe I was being unrealistic to think I could get through this thing without the trauma and side effects of the more conventional treatments. "After all," I thought, "I have one of the best urologists in the northeast, and he would be the expert in these matters."

I later discovered that other patients received similar responses from their urologists when asked about proton therapy. I also learned the sad fact that most general practitioners and urologists, at that time, were unfamiliar with proton technology. This is changing rapidly.

After replaying in my mind, the events of the meeting with my urologist, it started to become clear to me. He really couldn't answer my questions about proton therapy, because he really didn't know much about it. Yet a hospital in Southern California spent $100 million on this technology in the late 1980s and has treated thousands of patients over the past several years, apparently with excellent results. And, at least two other major medical centers, including Massachusetts General Hospital – right in my doctor's back yard – were building proton treatment centers. This treatment *had* to be a legitimate technology.

This was a major realization for me, and it reaffirmed my earlier conclusion that *I needed to take charge of my treatment decision.*

I couldn't leave this critical decision in the hands of my urologist – and no man should. I had lived my whole life believing that, "The doctor always knows best." And I learned during this journey, this isn't always true. Our doctors might, in good faith, feel they're making the best recommendation for us patients, but that's not always the case, *especially when it comes to treating prostate cancer.*

> *Tip: If you get nothing more from this book than this, it will have been worth your investment: Take charge of your treatment decision. Don't rely on your urologist alone. He or she is fundamentally a surgeon. That's what they know best and that's typically what they recommend. It may not be best for you. There are alternatives and each of them should be evaluated before you make your treatment decision.*

I had left my urologist's office even more confused and anxious than when I entered. But I found myself more determined than ever to continue my search for the *right* treatment for me.

The packet of information my urologist gave me included information about the surgical procedure, called radical prostatectomy, as well as some statistics on the "gold standard," as it is often called.

Among these papers was a consent form that described possible complications and side effects from surgery. These included the following:

- Impotence (inability to achieve or maintain an erection)

- Incontinence (inability to maintain urinary control)

- Strictures of bladder and/or urethra requiring stretching or further procedures

- Damage to rectal wall (requiring temporary colostomy)

- No guarantee of cancer cure

- Infection of incision requiring further treatment

- Emboli (blood clots) from veins into the lung (rare, serious)

At this point, I remember saying to my wife, "I think I'll continue my research."

CHAPTER 5

Understanding My Diagnosis

"Nothing in life is to be feared, it is only to be understood."
– Marie Curie

Cancer Grading and Staging

The next thing I needed to know was what the doctor meant by cancer stage and grade. And why should I feel good about having a T1c, Gleason 5 diagnosis?

Here is what I learned about the difference between stage and grade:

Grade describes how closely the individual cancer cells resemble normal cells of the same type, thus giving an indication of how fast the cancer is growing.

Stage describes the extent of the cancer in your body, or how far the cancer has spread.

Grading – Gleason Score

So, why should I feel good about a 3+2=5? I learned that biopsy samples are examined under a microscope by a pathologist. The shape and form of the cells are a clear indication of a pattern that indicates the level of aggressiveness of the cancer. Figure 5-1 shows what the pathologist sees under a microscope when he/she is looking at the five patterns, or levels, of prostate cancer.

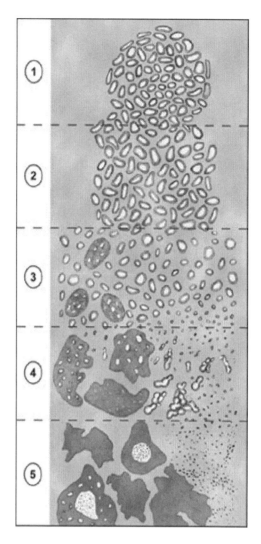

Fig. 5-1. Source: *American Journal of Surgical Pathology,* Volume 29, Number 9, September 2005. *The 2005 International Society of Urological Pathology (ISUP) Consensus Conference on Gleason Grading of Prostatic Carcinoma,* Jonathan Epstein, MD, William C. Allsbrook, Jr, MD, Mahul B. Admin, AD, and Lars Edgevad, MD, PhD, and the ISUP Grading Committee

46

Pattern 1. Well-differentiated cells that look similar to normal cells. These cells are typically round, closely packed and have well-defined edges.

Pattern 2. Still well-differentiated, but slightly less so than Pattern 1 cells. They are more loosely packed and may have less well-defined edges.

Pattern 3. Moderately differentiated. These may be medium sized cells, irregularly shaped, and not forming chains or cords.

Pattern 4. These are glands or cells of all sizes fused into cords or chains.

Pattern 5. Similar to pattern 4, but with large clear cancer cells.

The pathologist examines all the biopsy samples and scores each. He then takes the two most prominent Gleason patterns and adds them together – in my case 3+2, for a Gleason score of 5. The maximum Gleason score is 10 (5+5) and is indicative of the most aggressive cancer. Overall, Gleason scores in the 5 to 6 range are considered early stage or low grade. Scores in the 8 to 10 range imply advanced stage. My score of 5 put me at the low end of early stage.

A Gleason score of 3+2=5 has a dominant, moderately differentiated pattern (i.e., pattern 3) and a less dominant, well-differentiated pattern (i.e., pattern 2). A 4+3=7 Gleason score means that a poorly differentiated component (pattern 4) is dominant. If 95 percent or more of the tumor has the same characteristic pattern, then the same number is counted twice, example: 4+4=8.

New Development: Changes in Gleason Score Reporting

As mentioned above, when I was diagnosed in 2000, my first reported Gleason score was 3+2=5. I sought a second opinion on my slides from a different pathology lab and was told my score was 3+3=6. I was told this was not significant and that I should proceed with selecting a treatment option.

Tip: Always get a second opinion on your biopsy slides. This is a critically important step that will be explained in more detail later in this book.

Over the past few years there's been a shift away from the lower reported scores. As a result, you almost never see a Gleason score lower than 3+3=6. I assumed that, because of the subjectivity associated with reading pathology slides, pathologists around the world have agreed that if cancer is present, they would no longer report a Gleason score lower than 6. I was partly right.

Jonathan Epstein, M.D., at Johns Hopkins has the reputation of being one of the premier pathologists in the world. His lab is one of three recommended in the appendix of this book for a second opinion on pathology slides.

To get some clarification on this, I called Dr. Epstein's lab and spoke with Jeremy Miller, M.D. He confirmed that there has been a change in reporting of Gleason scores *from needle biopsies.* He told me that low grade – reported as Gleason score 2 to 4 – adenocarcinomas are often under-graded. The exception seems to be when the entire prostate is biopsied following radical prostatectomy, or when needle biopsy slides are read by expert urological pathologists. So, Dr. Epstein proposed, in an article he wrote for the *American Journal of Surgical Pathology* in 2000, that Gleason scores from needle biopsies no longer be reported below 5.

Later, in 2015, Dr. Epstein recommended, along with MJ Zelefsky and DD Sjoberg, in the *Journal of European Urology* (2015) that Gleason scores from needle biopsies no longer be reported below 3+3=6. Most medical centers seem to have adopted this practice. In recent years, I haven't heard of Gleason scores lower than 3+3=6.

This has led to the creation of a new problem: Now that the lowest Gleason score is assigned a 6 on a scale of 2-10, there's an incorrect assumption by many men that, since their cancer score is above the middle of the scale range, their cancer must be aggressive. Sadly, many doctors fail to tell their patients with Gleason score 6 that their grading is at the *bottom* of the *reported* range.

The fact that low Gleason scores are rarely seen does not mean that men are being diagnosed with more aggressive cancers. On the contrary – improvements in testing protocols are helping to find prostate cancers at earlier stages. This change in Gleason scoring reporting helps to prevent under-grading, and thus under-treating prostate cancer. Indolent (non-aggressive) cancers are frequently diagnosed, and these often need no treatment at all.

Second Pathology Report

Somewhere in my research I learned that a pathologist's reading of biopsy slides under a microscope is a subjective process, and it's a good idea to have your slides read by a second pathology lab. So, I called my urologist and made the request. He agreed that it was a wise move and sent my slides to another pathology lab in Boston.

A week later I was sorry I had made the request. The second lab read my slides as a 3+3, or Gleason score 6. This meant they felt my two most prominent patterns of cancer were at level 3. Now what? Which lab was right? Was I a Gleason 5 or 6? As it turns out, in this case it didn't really matter.

This experience taught me, however, the importance of getting a second opinion on your biopsy slides from another pathologist. Why? Because some differences might dictate different approaches to treating the cancer, or perhaps even cause you to rule out a particular treatment method. A Gleason 8 versus a Gleason 7, for example, could indicate a much higher probability of the cancer spreading beyond the gland. In this case, a patient may want to favor an approach that treats the entire prostate bed rather than the prostate gland alone.

Tip: Since the reading of biopsy slides is a subjective process, have your slides read by at least two laboratories. The appendix includes a listing of the premier pathology labs in the U.S.

Staging

I learned in my research that there are two commonly used staging systems – ABCD and TNM. The ABCD system has been used the longest, but is being replaced by the TNM staging system, which seems to be more commonly used. TNM staging is usually combined with a number such as 1, 2, or 3. The three letters T, N and M, respectively refer to the prostate *T*umor, the lymph *N*odes and *M*etastasis or distant spread of the disease.

ABCD Staging

Stage A cancers have no symptoms, and there is no detectable abnormality by DRE. Cancer is confined to the prostate and is accidentally discovered while surgery is being performed for other reasons.

Stage B cancers are usually discovered by needle biopsy that is done as a result of rising PSA or tumor felt by DRE.

Stage C cancer cells have spread outside the prostate capsule to the surrounding tissue and possibly the seminal vesicles, which are the glands that produce the semen.

Stage D cancer cells have spread or metastasized to lymph nodes, organs or tissue distant from the prostate. This could include the liver, bones or lungs.

TNM Staging

T1a is similar to Stage A, in that there are no symptoms and the cancer is accidentally discovered. These cancers are low grade and involve less than 5 percent of the tissue sampled

T1b is also similar to Stage A, but the cancer cells can be either low or high grade and involve more than 5 percent of the tissue sampled.

T1c was my cancer stage. This cancer is similar to Stage B. The tumor is detected by needle biopsy as a result of elevated PSA.

T2a cancer involves half of one lobe of the prostate, or less, and can be felt by DRE.

T2b cancer involves more than half of one lobe, but not both sides of the prostate.

T2c involves both lobes.

T3a is similar to Stage C and indicates that the cancer has spread beyond the capsule on one side of the gland.

T3b cancer has spread beyond the prostate capsule on both sides and involves the seminal vesicles.

T4 indicates that the cancer has spread into adjacent structures such as the bladder, levator muscles, pelvic wall or rectum.

NX Regional lymph nodes cannot be assessed

N0 No regional lymph node metastasis

N1 is similar to Stage D. Cancer cells have extended to a single pelvic lymph node 2 cm or less in size.

N2 cells are in a single pelvic lymph node greater than 2 cm in size

N3 cells have spread to any pelvic lymph node with more than 5 cm in greatest dimension.

M1 indicates distant metastasis to other parts of the body outside of the pelvic region.

Understanding this whole table is a little challenging at first. I settled on just understanding my own staging level, which was T1c, with no "N" and no "M," thank God. Again, my T1c indicated the cancer was discovered by needle biopsy that was performed as a result of rising PSA, and there was no palpable tumor – i.e. no tumor felt by DRE. The vast majority of diagnosed prostate cancers, I later discovered, fall into the T1/T2 category.

X-rays, Rads And Gray

Our next planned stop was with a radiation oncologist. But before that meeting, I had some more studying to do. I needed the answers to some questions: How does radiation kill cancer? What kind of radiation is used? How much radiation is necessary? Do they still use the term "Rads" to measure radiation as they did when I was in college? How do they prevent damage to healthy organs and tissues when bombarding my private parts with this deadly beam?

I didn't have answers to all these questions before the next appointment, but I expanded my knowledge in a couple of areas. I learned that X-ray radiation is also called "photon radiation," and that X-rays are a form of electromagnetic radiation, similar to radio waves and visible light, but with much shorter wavelength. X-rays, or photons, have no mass, and they travel at the speed of light. They interact electrically with atoms that make up the cells in our bodies, even though they have no net electrical charge.

The International System of Measurement (SI) has chosen the term Cobalt Gray, or more commonly, Gray (abbreviated "Gy") as the radiation unit of measurement. More correctly, the Gy is the unit of *absorbed* dose. One Gy is equivalent to 100 Rads, the term I was more familiar with from college physics.

Meeting with a Radiation Oncologist

Armed with this new information, my wife and I met with another Boston physician who specialized in conformal external beam radiation therapy (EBRT). Here I learned I was an "ideal candidate for EBRT" – a "poster boy," in fact. This was beginning to get interesting. How could I be the "poster boy" for both surgery and EBRT?

I began asking questions: How much radiation would I be receiving? What are my chances of survival? What is the probability of impotence, incontinence, rectal damage, and other side effects?

I learned that at that time, late 2000, they typically delivered about 75 Gy of photon (X-ray) radiation to the tumor site. I also learned that, in order to minimize collateral radiation damage to other parts of my body, they would be sending in the radiation beam from several angles around the perimeter of my pelvic region. I did a quick mental inventory of important body parts in my pelvic region, and I remember feeling nauseous.

"What about side effects?" I asked. "Short term, you might experience some urinary urgency, urinary burning and fatigue. The most common long-term side effects are impotence, incontinence and rectal damage. There could also be urethra strictures."

Noticing the beads of perspiration, loss of color, and panicked look on my face, the doctor smiled and told me that, because of my age and physical condition, I was unlikely to experience all these things. I'd probably come through this with only mild forms of these side effects. I remember thinking, "How can I be *mildly* incontinent? Maybe I'd need only two diapers a day instead of five?"

It was during this meeting that I realized I feared incontinence the most. True, I was only 57, and my wife and I still enjoyed regular intimacy. Certainly, the loss of sexual function would be terrible. But loss of bladder control, "That's what happens to old people," I thought, "in nursing homes!" I had 30 to 40 more years to live. I didn't want to spend that time in diapers. Could he guarantee I wouldn't be incontinent? "Sorry, but I can't," he said.

Brachytherapist Meeting

Gaining in knowledge (and new levels of fear), my wife and I next met with a prominent Boston oncologist who specialized in brachytherapy, or radioactive seed implants.

This physician told me I was an ideal candidate for seeds. And, in fact, considering my cancer stage, age, prostate size, and physical health, he said, "You're a perfect candidate for seeds." I remember commenting, "Would you say I'm the 'poster boy' for seeds?" He responded, "You could say that." Terrific, now I'm the poster boy for surgery, EBRT, and seeds. What more could I ask for?

He then described the procedure in detail and told me my chances for a cure were very good. The side effects, he explained were similar to those of EBRT, but with much less radiation exposure to my torso, since all the radiation would be coming from inside my prostate. He also told me about the possibility of seed migration, and that since I would be radioactive for a few months, I'd have to be careful about being near young children and pregnant women.

I took the opportunity of asking this doctor about proton therapy. He had some familiarity with this modality, but not a lot. He noted that protons are a type of radiation, and that radiation does, in fact, kill cancer, so, "It's probably a viable treatment option."

Before our meeting ended, I decided to confront this "poster boy" issue head on. "I have a question," I said, "I set you up earlier on this 'poster boy' issue. You're the third doctor who's told me I was the 'poster boy' for his treatment. How can I possibly be the 'poster boy' for surgery, EBRT and brachytherapy?" His answer was a revelation. He smiled and said, "Considering your age, cancer stage and physical health, whatever you choose for treatment, whether it be surgery, seeds, EBRT, cryotherapy, or proton radiation, it will most likely work for you – all with about the same, excellent chances of a cure. So, learn what you can about each option, especially side effects and quality-of-life issues, and choose the one that best meets your needs."

I felt a thousand-pound weight lifted from my shoulders. This took the pressure off surgery and gave me the incentive to keep all options on the table, and to crank up my research. My optimism was back.

CHAPTER 6

Investigating Treatment Options

"The more alternatives, the more difficult the choice."
– Abbe' D'Allanival

Now My Research Gets Serious

Where should I go to fill in the gaps, to find out more about the specifics of each option, and especially the dreaded side effects? Should I focus on books, the Internet, or word of mouth? I learned that all three would serve as important information sources, but nothing – it turned out – would be more valuable than my personal interviews with former patients.

Books and magazine articles are generally thoroughly researched, well organized, refined documentations about medical research and individual case histories. The quality of information is generally good, as publishers demand that quality work is distributed under their names. I read several books and journals on prostate cancer prevention, detection, and treatment.

I found the Internet rich with information on prostate cancer. Topics tend to be specific and the technology presented is usually current. For example, you can gather considerable information on something as specific as free PSA or the impact of diet and nutrition on prostate cancer prevention. There are also websites available where people can chat with others who are recently diagnosed patients, treated patients, or doctors involved in diagnosing and treating prostate cancer.

I spent days reading everything I could find about radical prostatectomy, all forms of external beam radiation therapy, brachytherapy (seed implant), cryosurgery (or cryoablation); as well as hormone treatment and watchful waiting (now called active surveillance).

Talk with the Customer

I have always been a believer in evaluating a product or service by checking with the customer. When making important investments in goods or services, I've always made it a point to check references, talking with customers who have used these goods and services. A happy customer speaks volumes about the quality and value of something in which you're about to make an investment. So, why shouldn't this work when evaluating prostate cancer treatment options?

Gaining access to former patients in some cases was a challenge at first, but my persistence and determination prevailed. Some of my best information came from interviewing men who had chosen different options.

Information I gathered in my research fills several boxes and a substantial portion of my computer hard drive. I won't attempt to regurgitate everything I learned in my research. Instead, I'll summarize the fundamentals in simple terms, and provide my assessment of the pros and cons of each option, much of which was influenced by my patient interviews.

Note: I have expanded this section to include my research on procedures that are now used, but were not readily available when I was doing my due diligence in late 2000

1. SURGERY (Radical Prostatectomy)

I frequently heard surgery referred to as the "Gold Standard" of prostate cancer treatments. It certainly has been the most common treatment option prescribed by doctors and chosen by patients over the years. The theory is that if the cancer is confined to the prostate and the gland is surgically removed, there's no chance for the cancer to spread to other parts of the body. This is true, but there are two major qualifiers here: 1) *If* the cancer is confined to the prostate, and 2) *If* no cancerous prostate tissue is left behind.

I would later learn there is reasonable probability, even for early stage cancer patients like me, that microscopic cancer cells have escaped the prostate gland. And when this happens, it usually "hangs around" the prostate capsule surface for some time before it eventually migrates to the lymph nodes and then is transmitted to other parts of the body (metastasis).

Radical prostatectomy is *major* surgery. It's one of the most challenging operations in urology. Surgery isn't suited for elderly men or men who are in poor or marginal physical condition. Men with certain heart problems, for example, might not want to subject themselves to the trauma of surgery.

Surgery can carry undesirable side effects including impotence and incontinence. Additionally, since the cancer is not always confined to the prostate, a certain percentage of patients who undergo this procedure require re-treatment when the cancer returns. The re-treatment usually involves one of the other treatment options (radiation, seeds, cryoablation, etc.).

I had firsthand knowledge of surgery, having observed my brother's case. Also, several friends and acquaintances had chosen surgery. I made it a point to speak with all of them.

From my research I learned that the procedure involved preparation, which often included banking a few pints of the patient's own blood over a period of several weeks. This was for the inevitable blood loss that accompanies major surgery (newer robotic techniques typically result in less blood loss). The patient is typically placed under general anesthesia. An intravenous tube is inserted in the arm to provide fluids until the patient is able to eat and drink. Oxygen is administered until blood oxygen level is normalized. And a small drain is placed in the incision to remove fluid following surgery.

The prostate is located deep within the pelvis and is surrounded by organs and structures that are vulnerable to injury. This includes the bladder, the rectum and nerve bundles that are essential for male potency. An incision is made between the penis and navel. Next, a major vein system is carefully severed, and the urethra is cut making sure not to damage the urethral sphincter that controls urination.

The doctor then makes the decision as to how much, if any, of the nerve bundles that surround the prostate can be spared. It's these nerve bundles that control erectile function. The surgeon next separates the prostate from the bladder and removes the seminal vesicles and surrounding tissue. Finally, the doctor reattaches the bladder and urethra and begins the process of suturing up the patient.

During the procedure, a catheter is inserted into the penis in order to drain urine from the bladder. The catheter remains in place for about two weeks.

Recuperation from surgery generally takes from one to three months. During that time the patient must deal with bowel issues, catheter management and removal, and temporary incontinence.

Cure rates with all forms of treatment vary by cancer stage and many other factors. Certainly younger, healthier men with early stage prostate cancer will experience higher cure rates than average.

A June 2008 article in the *Journal of the American Medical Association* (JAMA) by Patrick Walsh, M.D. and several other physicians at Johns Hopkins reports, "Although surgery provides excellent cancer control, approximately 15 to 40 percent of these men will experience cancer recurrence within 5 years."

Most of the men I interviewed told me they had no regrets for having chosen surgery, although several said things like, "I hope I'll never have to go through something like that again." A few were incontinent, or marginally continent, and most seemed reluctant to talk about impotence. Sexual potency is something we males equate to our "manhood," and thus, when it diminishes, we aren't always honest about our status. Those who admitted to impotence seemed to be split into two groups. One group was completely impotent with erectile dysfunction and no libido. The other group used medications (e.g. Viagra), devices (pumps), injections, or implants with varying degrees of success.

Because men are reluctant to talk about loss of sexual potency, I suspect the impotency numbers reported for *all* treatment options are understated.

While most of the surgery patients I interviewed seemed to be doing well, three had experienced relapses, and had undergone follow-up salvage treatments, including radiation and/or hormone therapy. One had a urethral stricture resulting from his surgery and had to undergo a "Roto-Rooter procedure" as he described it. One experienced an infection that caused much discomfort for weeks following surgery. Another told me of an acquaintance who had surgery and had serious complications from blood clots.

I really didn't want to have surgery, and my interviews helped with my decision.

Here Is What I Learned Are the Advantages of Surgery:

- Surgery is called the "Gold Standard" because it's the oldest and most common treatment for prostate cancer. There is more statistical data available on cure rates and side effects for surgery than any other treatment option.

- For some men, there's a psychological benefit knowing the cancerous gland has been removed from their body.

- *If* the cancer is confined to the prostate and if no cancerous tissue is left behind, the cancer is gone for good.

And the Disadvantages of Surgery:

- Surgery requires hospitalization. A radical prostatectomy is *major* surgery, which means trauma and probable blood loss.

- Risks from anesthesia, especially for older adults, can include postoperative confusion, pneumonia, stroke and heart attack.

- Risk of infection with any surgery, especially one as invasive as a radical prostatectomy

- Risk of death. Though rare, one "side effect" rarely discussed between doctor and patient is the risk of death from prostate surgery. *The Journal of the National Cancer Institute* reports a 0.5 percent risk of death within 30 days of prostate surgery (that's one in 200) for men up to age 69, and up to 1.1 percent (one in 100) for men 70 and older.

- There's a long recuperation period following surgery – usually two or three months before full physical activity can be resumed. Fatigue sometimes lasts for a year or more.

- Surgery carries a 50 to 85 percent chance of erectile dysfunction or impotence. Most literature reports a 75 percent chance of impotency, or three out of four men. Nerve sparing surgeons report impotence statistics in the 10 to 25 percent range, but many doubt the validity of these claims. Age, general health, and the experience of the surgeon are all important factors. A Swedish study reported, at the 2014 AUA annual meeting, that 84 percent of men experienced erectile dysfunction after surgery (see bibliography).

- Urinary incontinence occurs in 20 to 40 percent of the cases. Patient age and the physician's skills are important factors. After three years these numbers can drop to as low as 10 percent according to the *Prostate Cancer Foundation.*

- About 5 percent of men will require follow-up surgery to correct incontinence issues according to a study reported in *Reuters* on July 2, 2012.

- Loss of ejaculate, since the prostate, which supplies the bulk of the fluid has been removed.

- Other less common side effects are strictures of the bladder or urethra, damage to the rectal wall, blood clots and increased risk of inguinal hernias.

- An article in the *New England Journal of Medicine*, Vol. 346, No. 15, April 2002, reported:

  o 0.4 to 0.9 percent surgery related deaths
  o Postoperative complications, 29-35 percent
  o Late urinary complications 25-28 percent, Major events 17-19 percent
  o Long term incontinence 18-24 percent. Major events 7-9 percent.

- Penis shrinkage. It's been reported that the penis will shrink from one-half to one inch in length from radical prostatectomy. This is probably a result of reattaching the urethra to the bladder after the prostate has been removed. It may also have something to do with scarring from the procedure. *Men's Health* reports, "The average reported loss among the men was one centimeter – or about one-third of an inch. But some patients came through surgery missing nearly an inch and a half from their former expanse, a separate study found." It's been reported that much of the loss is recovered over time.

- Surgery often removes the tumor incompletely, leaving cancer in the margins. A positive margin occurs in 11 – 48 percent of surgical cases.

- Surgery has little value if the cancer has progressed beyond the prostate. This microscopic cancer usually cannot be seen at the time of surgery. If found later, it requires follow-up salvage treatment.

- Surgery is heavily practitioner dependent. Many urologists claim to do "nerve-sparing surgery." But doctors, with different levels of experience, using different techniques, have a broad range of results. Despite what some physicians say, a radical prostatectomy is not "routine surgery."

Tip: Thousands of urologists do radical prostatectomies every day. The operation is serious and delicate. Not all doctors employ the same techniques. Many doctors claim to do "nerve-sparing surgery," implying that they make every attempt to save the nerve bundles necessary for sexual function. Be sure to check out the doctor who will perform your surgery. How many procedures has he or she done? Speak with 10 to 15 men who have been operated on by this surgeon. What have been their results and side effects? Choose only the most experienced and successful doctor for this complex and invasive procedure.

Laparoscopic Surgery

An alternative to "open prostate surgery" as described above is laparoscopic radical prostatectomy (LRP). When the first edition of

61

this book was published in 2006, this procedure was relatively new, quite complex and not very common. Louis Kavoussi, a pioneering laparoscopic surgeon, who is vice chairman of urology at Johns Hopkins Medical Center, performed 20 of these procedures and stopped, because he didn't think the operation, which took an average of nine hours, was superior to open surgery.

Since then, the newer DaVinci laparoscopic robotic surgical technique has grown in popularity and use. DaVinci laparoscopic robotic surgery typically involves less blood loss and results in shorter recovery times, but side effects, it appears, are still comparable to open surgery and may be even worse. This has been borne out in published literature and our own patient interviews.

Robotic-assisted surgery also requires considerable skill and experience by the doctor in order to be safe and effective. According to an article in *Bloomberg News*, researchers reported more than 1,600 procedures need to be done before the surgeon is proficient and able to remove all the malignant cells in the prostate bed.

A study published in 2009 compared data from the *National Cancer Institute's* SEER Medicare database involving 1,938 men who underwent robotic surgery to 6,899 men who underwent open surgery. The robotic surgery group had shorter hospital stays (two days vs. three days) far fewer blood transfusions and a lower risk of respiratory and other surgical complications. But they also had more than twice the risk of genitourinary complications, a 30 percent increased risk of incontinence and a 40 percent increased risk of erectile dysfunction 18 months after the procedure.

If you are seriously considering DaVinci laparoscopic robotic surgery, be sure to question your doctor's level of experience with this technique. *The New York Times* reported on March 25, 2013 that an inexperienced surgeon performed DaVinci laparoscopic robotic surgery on a 67-year-old man leaving him "incontinent and with a colostomy bag, and leading to kidney and lung damage, sepsis and a stroke." He survived his injuries but died sometime later, from complications related to his surgery.

While laparoscopic robotic surgery is gaining in popularity, because it generally involves less blood loss and results in shorter recovery times, the complications can sometimes be more severe. Rectal injury, for example, is more common with the laparoscopic procedure, according to an article in *Newsweek* magazine. *The*

Journal of Clinical Oncology reported that while robotic surgery is likely to result in less blood loss and faster recovery than traditional open surgery, the most feared of all – incontinence and sexual impotence – "are high after both."

Bert Vorstman, BSc, MD, MS, FAAP, FRACS, FACS, reports in a recent article (see references in appendix), "From death within 30 days of surgery to suicidal depression and deep vein thrombosis, many other general surgical complications have been recorded" (i.e. side effects experienced with both open surgery and robotic surgery). He further states, "As well, there are complications specific to robotic surgery such as insufflation embolism, trocar injuries and positioning injuries and, injuries that are particular to prostate removal itself."

Finally, an important article based on a study at Duke University was published in *The New York Times*, Aug. 27, 2008, titled "Regrets after Prostate Surgery." The article notes that, "One in five men who undergoes prostate surgery to treat cancer later regrets the decision," and men who elected robotic surgery, "were four times more likely to regret their choice than men who had undergone the open procedure."

Tip: This reinforces my belief that "checking with the customer," i.e. one who has been through any treatment option you are considering, is essential to making the right treatment decision for yourself.

2. EXTERNAL BEAM RADIATION THERAPY

Through my research and conversations with radiation oncologists I learned several interesting things about radiation and cancer:

1. Radiation has been used to kill cancer for about 100 years.
2. Urologists are reluctant to operate on men older than 69 or 70 (for good reason) – and radiation is usually the treatment of choice in these cases.
3. Radiation is often prescribed for men with health issues that might be compromised or exacerbated by the trauma of surgery.
4. Radiation is commonly used as a salvage treatment when surgery fails.

5. Radiation is a standard treatment for "localized" (non-metastasized) prostate cancer. This typically includes stages T1 through T3, or A, B and C.
6. The higher the radiation dose, the better the chance of a cure.

All forms of radiation kill cancer the same way – they permanently damage the cancer cell's DNA structure. The cells live out their "normal" life span, but the radiation damage prevents them from growing and dividing, and they eventually die off. This phenomenon is referred to as programmed cell death, or "apoptosis."

There are different forms of radiation, both in physical characteristics and in method of delivery to the cancer. I learned it's important to understand these differences since the impact on quality of life following treatment varies depending on the type of radiation and the method of delivery.

The four types of radiation used to kill cancer are X-rays (or photons), protons, gamma rays, and neutrons. Gamma rays and neutrons are seldom used, so I'm focusing on just two: X-rays (photons) and protons.

It's important to understand the fundamental difference between these two types of radiation. In simplest terms, X-ray (photon) radiation is at its maximum intensity where it *enters* the body at the surface of the skin. It loses energy on the way to the tumor site, thus radiating everything in its path as it travels *into* the body, passing through the target tumor site and then *out* of the body. For this reason, multiple body entry points must be selected to reduce collateral damage to healthy tissue and organs.

Proton radiation is quite different. It loses a small portion of its energy on the way to the tumor site, deposits the bulk of its energy on the target volume (e.g. the prostate), and has a zero exit dose. This results in significantly less radiation deposited on healthy tissues and organs.

Radiation treatment is painless, tasteless, and has no smell. Radiation treatment goals can be either palliative (to improve the quality of life in a patient with terminal or irreversible cancer) or curative (to attempt to cure or rid a patient of his/her cancer). My research focused on the latter.

Conventional External Beam Radiation

Conventional external beam radiation therapy (EBRT) involves directing high-energy photons (X-rays) to the cancer site.

Instead of administering all the radiation in one dose, which would cause serious, irreparable harm to the patient, it's delivered in small "fractions" over an extended period of time. Each treatment lasts only a few minutes and is painless. The entry point of the radiation is usually varied in order to minimize damage to healthy tissue. The challenge with all forms of radiation is delivering maximum dosage to the cancer site without damaging surrounding healthy tissue and organs.

Common to all forms of external beam radiation is the planning process. It is important to precisely pinpoint the treatment target volume and plan the treatment series. In treating prostate cancer, physicians typically prescribe about 40 treatments. Treatment sessions usually last about 15 to 20 minutes, once a day, five days a week.

Three-Dimensional Conformal Radiation Therapy (3D-CRT)

As the name implies, this method of delivering photons involves the use of computers to accurately map the prostate area. The patient is immobilized, and radiation is delivered from multiple angles. The radiation beam is shaped to include a three-dimensional anatomic configuration of the prostate. The intent with conformal radiation therapy is to target the tumor volume more precisely and to reduce damage to surrounding organs and tissue. 3D-CRT allows higher doses of radiation to the prostate, with less normal tissue complications than conventional EBRT. This form of radiation therapy is diminishing in use, in favor of the more advanced IMRT.

Intensity Modulated Radiation Therapy (IMRT)

IMRT is an advanced form of 3D radiation therapy using X-ray (photon) radiation. Other forms of photon radiation use a single radiation beam of fixed energy level. IMRT varies the energy level over the field being treated by using multiple beams of varying intensity. The higher-intensity beams are directed at the thicker part of the tumor volume, and the lower intensity beams are aimed at thinner segments. Specialized equipment costing about $1 million is required to administer this treatment. Because it is more precisely focused, IMRT reduces the amount of radiation exposure to surrounding healthy tissue, and reportedly produces fewer side effects than EBRT or 3D-CRT.

IGRT

Image Guided Radiation Therapy (IGRT), an advanced form of IMRT, refers to imaging the prostate in the treatment room each day before the IMRT is delivered. Proponents feel that this ensures that the IMRT beam is aimed correctly every day. This image guidance may be through the use of gold fiducials (marker seeds) implanted in the prostate and imaged with low-dose orthogonal X-rays before each treatment, or by daily CT scan, where gold fiducials are not required.

RapidArc a form of Volumetric Modulated Arc Therapy (VMAT)

RapidArc is an advanced form of IMRT. Instead of treating from a limited number of fields as is done with IMRT, RapidArc treats continuously in a 360-degree circle (arc) around the patient, delivering radiation, literally from every angle.

To maximize precision, computers continuously vary the speed of the gantry, the shape of the aperture and the dose of the radiation. This helps to reduce the amount of radiation deposited on healthy organs and tissue.

It's important to note, however, that RapidArc technology is still based on conventional X-ray (photon) radiation, which means that everything in the 360-degree arc is being radiated as the beam enters and leaves the body. Theoretically this should produce fewer side effects than the other forms of X-ray radiation therapy mentioned above. But, as of this writing there is minimal data available on RapidArc and no substantive studies comparing these treatment modalities and toxicity (side effect) levels.

Other Forms of IMRT

Periodically, a radiation technology is developed that has some small variation over previous technologies. It's typically given a new name and then the marketing begins. TomoTherapy®, for example is another form of IMRT that uses CT scanning technology for image guidance. Other types of IMRT are sure to surface as technology develops, particularly newer imaging technologies.

Tumor Targeting in the Future?

Physicians are considering the possibility of using daily imaging techniques to focus on the tumor within the prostate and not treat the entire prostate. This is quite controversial, as microscopic prostate cancer cells may not be visible, even to advanced imaging techniques, and therefore missed in daily treatment.

Stereotactic Body Radiation Therapy (SBRT)

This external beam radiation technique uses advanced image guidance to deliver large doses of radiation to the target volume (prostate). And because each dose is significantly higher than the other treatment options, the entire course of treatment lasts only a few days, usually five.

Different types of SBRT include Gamma Knife®, S-Knife®, Clinac® and the most common, CyberKnife®, which we will cover here.

CyberKnife

CyberKnife is an advanced form of photon (X-ray) radiotherapy. Its primary use in the past has been in treating head and brain tumors, but it's also being used to treat tumors in other parts of the body including the prostate.

CyberKnife uses image guidance and computer-controlled robotics to compensate for patient movement throughout the treatment process. Live radiographic images are compared to pre-treatment CT or MRI scans to determine patient and tumor position throughout the course of treatment. For this reason, it is not necessary to use radiographic (e.g. gold seed) markers or fiducials.

CyberKnife is considered by some to be superior to IMRT because IMRT registers target location only at the beginning of each treatment, while CyberKnife continuously tracks the target location.

Practitioners believe that because they can more precisely target the tumor in real time, they can deliver higher doses per fraction (8-25 Gy, vs. about 2 Gy for other forms of radiotherapy). This allows physicians to reduce the total number of treatments – for prostate cancer, for example – from about 40, for other radiotherapies, to as few as five treatments.

According to the American Cancer Society (ACS), "The main advantage of SBRT over IMRT is that the treatment takes less time (days instead of weeks). The side effects, though, are not better. There is no long-term data on SBRT on disease-free survival, side effects or secondary cancers. And, some preliminary research has shown that certain side effects may be worse with SBRT than with IMRT."

Conventional (X-ray or Photon) Radiation Summary

For all practical purposes, IMRT and its various "cousins" represent the vast majority of X-ray (or photon) radiotherapies that are used today. There are some variations in each type of IMRT, but there are more similarities than differences.

SBRT, on the other hand is quite different, in that significantly higher doses of radiation are administered over just a few days. Very little data is available on SBRT (CyberKnife) results, and the following commentary on advantages, disadvantages and side effects apply only to the IMRT options.

Tip: IGRT, Tomotherapy and RapidArc are all forms of IMRT. They are often marketed as the latest and most advanced forms of radiotherapy. Some physicians feel these forms of IMRT are superior to basic IMRT, and others do not. It seems that those who have the specialized equipment promote their technology as the most advanced and the best for treating prostate cancer.

But the studies haven't been done. One thing all oncologists and physicists agree on is this: The less radiation deposited on healthy tissue, and the more deposited on the tumor volume, the better it is for the patient.

Advantages of Radiation Therapy:

- Data suggests, the long-term cure rates for all forms of external beam radiation are equivalent to surgery.
- External radiation therapy is noninvasive. There's no pain, trauma or blood loss during treatment.
- Hospitalization is not required. Treatment is done on an out-patient basis.

Disadvantages of Radiation Therapy:

- Eight to nine weeks of treatment are typically necessary to safely deliver all the radiation necessary to kill the cancer. But this is changing and will be explained later in this book.
- The literature reports 30 to 60 percent of the patients who choose external beam radiation therapy experience some degree of sexual dysfunction after completing treatment. Although this figure is high, it's generally lower than the surgical alternative. Age, general health and the specific radiation treatment chosen all affect this outcome.
- Urinary incontinence has been reported in 5 to 20 percent of cases, again depending on many factors.
- Radiation proctitis can occur in some cases resulting in diarrhea, blood in the stool and rectal leakage. Most of these problems go away over time.
- Bladder irritation can result in temporary urinary burning or blood in the urine. These issues usually go away over time.
- Erection problems, including impotence can occur. The American Cancer Society states that "After a few years, the impotence rate after radiation is about the same as that after surgery. Problems with erections usually do not occur right after radiation therapy, but slowly develop over time. This is

69

different from surgery, where impotence occurs immediately and may get better over time."

- Because many more fields are treated with IMRT, and because of the nature of X-ray radiation, the amount of radiation deposited on healthy organs and tissue is high with this form of radiotherapy. This can result in collateral damage, including secondary cancers later in life.
- Short-term side effects from external beam radiation may include fatigue and possibly skin irritation.
- A less common side effect is a urethral stricture, which might require treatment to remove the obstruction.

Tip: The term "incontinence" is often used to describe anything ranging from minimal leakage to complete loss of bladder control. When you're talking with a doctor or interviewing a former patient, be sure you understand what they mean by the term, "incontinence." For example, some men I interviewed reported they were not incontinent, but later admitted to wearing pads while sleeping or leaking during physical exertion. Others said they experienced "stress incontinence," or loss of urine during physical activity, such as coughing, sneezing, laughing or exercising.

3. BRACHYTHERAPY (Radioactive Seeds)

This technique involves delivering radiation to the tumor site from *within* the prostate. I learned that if I chose this option, a physician would surgically implant 50 to 125 tiny radioactive seeds directly into my prostate gland. These seeds emit low levels of radiation from a few weeks to several months, depending on the type of seeds used.

The patient is given a spinal or general anesthesia, and hollow needles containing the seeds are inserted into the prostate through the perineum, the area between the scrotum and the anus. Different imaging techniques are used by doctors to place the rice-sized seeds in the proper position within the gland.

The procedure takes two to three hours to perform. A catheter is inserted through the penis to drain the bladder, and the patient typically spends one night in the hospital. The next day, the catheter is removed, and the patient goes home. Pain and discomfort are nominal, and the patient usually resumes normal activities in a few days. Follow-up visits to the hospital are required for several weeks.

Because of the short treatment time, minimal trauma and rapid recovery, brachytherapy is gaining in popularity, particularly among younger men whose busy work schedules would be disrupted by the alternative treatment options.

A newer form of brachytherapy called Temporary High Dose Rate (or HDR) brachytherapy is available. This wasn't widely available when I was diagnosed, but is becoming more commonplace, especially as a treatment for recurrent prostate cancer. This technique uses higher doses of radiation from Iridium-192 or Cesium-137 seeds that are left in place for a short time (less than one hour) and then removed. Hollow needles deposit the seeds, which are in nylon tubes, through the perineum. The sleeves stay in place for 10 to 15 minutes. This is typically repeated one or two more times within two weeks of the initial treatment.

HDR brachytherapy is sometimes combined with external beam radiation to treat moderately aggressive to very aggressive localized prostate cancer.

Advantages of Brachytherapy:

- Cure rates comparable to surgery and external beam radiation options.
- Short hospitalization stay and quick recuperation period.
- Although it's a surgical procedure, brachytherapy is significantly less invasive than surgery. Trauma is minimal and there's essentially no blood loss.
- Since the radiation source is within the prostate gland, there's generally less radiation damage to other organs and tissue.

Disadvantages of Standard Brachytherapy (seeds left in place):

- Risks associated with spinal or general anesthesia.
- Risk of impotence and incontinence is comparable to external radiation.

- Higher risk of Grade 3 GU (genitourinary) morbidity (side effects), than with other forms of radiotherapy. Grade 3 morbidity is defined as, "Frequency with urgency and nocturia hourly or more frequently; dysuria, pelvis pain or bladder spasm requiring regular, frequent narcotic; gross hematuria with/without clot passage."
- Since the seeds remain in place indefinitely, they continue to emit low levels of radiation for several weeks to months. For this reason, patients are advised not to have close contact with pregnant women or young children for a few months.
- It's common for seeds to dislodge and migrate to other parts of the body including the lungs. The long-term impact of this is not known.
- Uncertainty as to whether sufficient dosage will reach the periphery of the gland where tumor recurrence/spread tends to occur.
- Initial training in this procedure was somewhat limited and standardization was lacking.
- Seeds can be passed in the semen to a partner during intercourse.
- One nuclear radiation expert has reported that during the first few weeks following seed implant, the patient may trigger highly sensitive terrorist alarms at airports.

There is conflicting information on brachytherapy side effects. Most of the literature seems to indicate that side effects are comparable to external beam radiation therapy. However, according to a study conducted by Dr. Jeff Michalski, assistant professor of radiation oncology at the Washington University School of Medicine, "Patients who underwent brachytherapy reported significantly more urinary, sexual and bowel problems than men treated with external-beam radiation."

An article in the *Journal of Urology* cited incontinence levels of up to 45 percent following brachytherapy.

On the subject of seed migration, the *Journal of Urology* (Urology 2002; 59:555-559) reported that with brachytherapy, in approximately 36 percent of the cases, a small number of radioactive seeds became dislodged and migrated to the lungs. Other studies have reported brachytherapy seeds migrating to the coronary artery. And,

72

while there is no evidence of short-term harm, the long-term effects are not known. Some work has been done to string seeds together to prevent migration, but little is known of the success of the technique at this writing.

The urethra, which channels urine and semen outside the body, runs through the center of the prostate gland. The center of the gland receives a much higher dose of radiation with brachytherapy, than with any other form of radiation therapy. This may be the reason for higher levels of urinary problems reported with brachytherapy.

The most important thing I learned about brachytherapy is that it's extremely practitioner dependent. Precise seed placement is critical. "Cold spots" between poorly placed seeds within the prostate, in the margins, and near the rectum (to reduce rectal side effects) can result in cancer recurrence. A small number of physicians who use advanced imaging techniques, and do a large number of procedures, have significantly better results than the others.

Tip: A growing number of doctors are performing this relatively new procedure. Precise placement of the radioactive seeds is the key to success. Different visualization and placement techniques are used by different doctors. If you choose this procedure, select one of the few doctors who use the most up-to-date technology and have done hundreds of procedures. Do your homework!

Brachytherapy cannot be performed on men with significantly enlarged prostates and is usually limited to stage A and B (T1, T2) cancers.

Andy Grove and Brachytherapy

Andy Grove was president and CEO of Intel, a man of considerable intellect and financial means. While surfing the Internet, I came across an article in *Fortune* magazine about his journey with prostate cancer. Grove had chosen hormones plus high dose rate brachytherapy (HDR) plus EBRT and wrote a comprehensive article on his diagnosis and treatment in the May 13, 1996, issue of *Fortune*.

The *Fortune* article was four years old when I found it, so I boldly decided to reach out to Mr. Grove to see what information I could gather from his experience. I called Intel corporate headquarters in Santa Clara, CA, and asked for Mr. Grove's office. His secretary ran interference and asked about the nature of my call. I told her my story and said that I had a few questions for Mr. Grove. She suggested I email him and gave me his email address.

In my first email, I indicated that I understood he is a high-profile person, and that I wouldn't reveal to others any personal or potentially embarrassing information that he shared with me. I listed several questions on the email, including some very personal questions about the common side effects of the treatment.

His response was prompt, and surprisingly frank and detailed. I had more questions, so I sent more emails. He answered all my questions frankly and honestly.

I continued my research into this form of treatment by tracking down and interviewing men who had chosen the brachytherapy option. I spoke with a few "conventional" brachytherapy patients but was unable to find others who had chosen the high-dose option. I suspect it's because HDR brachytherapy, especially in combination with EBRT, wasn't widely used at the time.

Two interesting anecdotes came out of my interviews with brachytherapy patients. The first involved a lawyer from New York. I received his name from one of his acquaintances. The lawyer agreed to speak with me on the condition that I keep his name confidential. I agreed and asked why. He told me that he was recently divorced and had two children and a new girlfriend. He said none of them knew of his diagnosis. He didn't want to frighten his kids or scare away his girlfriend. He also didn't want his law firm partners to know.

After he was diagnosed, he conducted his research and chose brachytherapy. Secretly, he scheduled his seed-implant treatment for a Friday afternoon and was back to work on the following Monday. When I spoke with him, which was two years later, his family, friends, and partners were unaware of his diagnosis and treatment.

Certainly, if someone can "bounce back" so quickly following a valid, proven treatment for prostate cancer, it was something that warranted serious consideration.

While I was doing my research, I received a call from a gentleman who heard I was evaluating prostate cancer treatment alternatives, and that I was interviewing former patients. He happened to be an attorney as well and was primarily focused on brachytherapy because of the minimal disruption to his lifestyle. I brought him up to date on my findings.

He asked if I could provide him the names of those I interviewed who had chosen brachytherapy. I gave him five names, and told him that I had a sixth name, a very well-informed gentleman who was a New York attorney, who asked me to keep his information confidential. He pleaded with me to get permission to talk with this gentleman. So, I emailed the first lawyer, gave him the name, address, phone number, and email address of the second lawyer, and encouraged him to call.

A week went by and I received an email from the first lawyer. He told me that coincidentally, the lawyer I referred to him was on the opposite side of a major legal battle on a very contentious case. However, under the circumstances, he called the second lawyer, shared his story, offered advice, and the two became friends – outside the courtroom. This certainly dispels one myth. Lawyers do have a heart – at least sometimes.

The one troubling thing my interviews of former brachytherapy patients revealed was lack of bladder control following treatment. About one in five reported varying levels of incontinence.

I concluded from my research that brachytherapy was a sound and viable treatment choice with its own unique set of advantages and disadvantages. And, if I were to go this route, my most important job was going to be to pick the right physician.

Recent Developments

One radiation oncologist who reviewed this latest edition pointed out the fact that the use of strands (or sleeves) can mitigate the seed migration issue with brachytherapy. He also noted there is a recent evolution in brachytherapy called MRI-Assisted Radiosurgery (MARS) that is attracting much attention. This bears looking into.

4. PROTON TREATMENT

Technically speaking, proton therapy is a form of external beam radiation therapy and it is image guided. But there are so many differences with this technology, due to the unique nature of the proton particle, it needs to be discussed separately.

As mentioned earlier, it's a widely known fact that radiation kills cancer. The more common form of radiation uses photons (X-rays) to attack the cancer. Photons begin to do their damage the instant they contact the body, and they give up that energy as they penetrate the body on the way to the tumor. After the photon radiation reaches the tumor and damages the DNA, it continues to move through the body, losing energy while passing through healthy cells as it exits the body.

Protons are sub-atomic particles, yet they're the largest particles in the atom. As such, they exhibit a unique characteristic called the *Bragg Peak*. The Bragg Peak refers to the proton beam's ability to pass into the body at high speed, travel to the location of the cancer deep within the body, and then release 90 percent of its cancer-killing energy *right on the target tumor volume*. Only 10 percent of the energy is deposited on healthy tissue on the way to the tumor. Once the energy is released at the tumor site, there's *no* exit dose, and therefore, *no* radiation exposure to healthy tissue and organs on the far side of the tumor. This unique characteristic – very low entrance dose and zero exit dose – represents *the major difference* from conventional photon/X-ray radiation, including IMRT, which dumps the *bulk* of its radiation energy on healthy tissue.

The figure below shows graphically how proton radiation differs from photon (X-ray) radiation. The target tumor is represented by the dark gray shaded area and is about 18 to 26 cm deep inside the male torso. The solid line shows what happens when photons (X-rays) enter the body. As you can see, photon radiation is at its maximum intensity as it enters the body radiating everything in its path. After it passes through the tumor, it continues to deposit radiation on healthy tissue as it leaves the body.

The dashed line represents proton radiation, which enters the body delivering significantly less radiation to healthy tissue. After reaching the target tumor, the proton radiation intensity drops to zero, minimizing radiation delivery to healthy tissue. So, with proton therapy, most of the cancer-killing radiation is deposited on the target tumor, and not healthy tissue. The result is destruction of the tumor while minimizing the probability of side effects or secondary cancers later in life.

76

**Proton vs. X-rays (Photons)
Comparing Healthy Tissue Radiation Exposure**

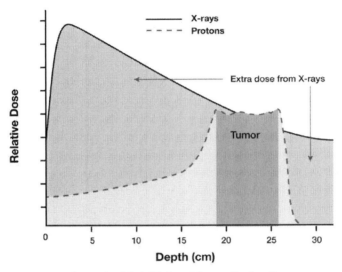

Image by Mark Hickey, Marcus Design Group

A recent study reported in JAMA Oncology, Nov. 25, 2019, titled, *Comparative Effectiveness of Proton vs Proton Therapy as Part of Concurrent Chemoradiotherapy for Locally Advanced Cancer,* did not focus on prostate cancer, but it did show the distinct benefits of the proton beam vs. photon technology in treating a variety of advanced, localized cancers reporting: "a two-thirds reduction in adverse events associated with unplanned hospitalizations, with no difference in disease-free or overall survival," as well as a significant reduction in severe adverse events compared with photon therapy, with comparable oncologic outcomes."

Once again, because of the unique characteristics of the proton beam, physicians can focus most of the cancer-killing radiation on the tumor target while minimizing radiation to surrounding healthy organs and tissues.

World-renowned radiation oncologist, Dr. Carl Rossi reported in the *Prostate Cancer Communication Newsletter* (Vol 23, No. 1

March 2007): "From a practical standpoint, the 'integral dose' (total dose to normal tissue) in a proton beam treatment plan for prostate cancer is **three** **to** **five** **times** *less* (emphasis added) than which is common when sophisticated X-ray therapy plans (utilizing IMRT) are employed."

Tip: No amount of radiation is good for healthy tissue Any treatment option that reduces radiation exposure to healthy tissue is fundamentally superior.

Carpet Bombing vs. Smart Bombing

Technologies have been developed that allow the proton beam to be precisely shaped in three dimensions and delivered to a site – such as the prostate – with extreme precision. One might look at conventional photon/X-ray radiation as "carpet bombing" which destroys the target, but also does widespread damage around a target site. Proton radiation, on the other hand is more like a "smart bomb" that precisely destroys the targets (tumor volume) while doing minimal to no collateral damage to nearby healthy organs and tissue. *This critical factor is extremely important when it comes to potential side effects and "quality-of-life" issues following treatment.*

Once again, according to Carl Rossi, M.D., in *Prostate Cancer Communication Newsletter*, Vol.23, No.1:

The rationale and desire to treat with protons is based on their physical superiority to X-rays. Simply put, a proton beam will stop at some point within the body, while X-rays will not. From a clinical standpoint, this unique aspect of proton beam radiation allows the radiation oncologist to reduce the normal tissue radiation dose to levels which are not possible with any type of X-ray therapy (including Intensity-Modulated Radiation Therapy and Tomotherapy) while simultaneously escalating the radiation dose to the target tumor.

Positioning the Patient

When I was diagnosed and doing my due diligence, there was only one proton center in the U.S., and it was located at the Loma Linda University Cancer Center in Southern California. As of this writing, there are 34 proton centers in the U.S. as you will learn later in this book. There are many similarities in these centers, in terms of how the proton particles are generated, accelerated, focused and delivered. There are also several differences. The following relates mostly to the Loma Linda process and procedures.

Since proton beam radiation is so precisely targeted, the patient must be placed in the exact same position for each treatment. Customized devices must be designed and built for each patient to allow the proton radiation to conform, three-dimensionally, to the target site.

In order to receive this treatment at Loma Linda, where I was treated, one must have a custom-fit immobilization pod, a half-pipe-shaped device that is used to precisely position the patient daily for the eight weeks of treatment. A CT scan is then done to produce a three-dimensional image of the prostate and surrounding area. This information is used to plan the treatment protocol.

Treatment begins with the insertion of a small balloon-type device in the rectum, which is filled with a small amount of water to "inflate" the rectum. The balloon serves two purposes: It ensures the bulk of the rectal wall is out of range of the radiation beam, and it helps to immobilize the prostate.

The patient lies in the pod and is positioned in the center of a specially designed, 100-ton, three-story-tall gantry. The customized focusing devices are attached to the machinery in the gantry, and the beam is delivered.

The treatment is painless and beam delivery takes about one minute; however, preparation and safety protocols extend the total time in the treatment room to about 15 minutes.

A Recent Advancement: A recently developed hydrogel product called, SpaceOAR is growing in popularity. Like the rectal balloon, this product is intended to protect the rectum from radiation damage. SpaceOAR is injected through the perineum (space between the anus and testes) and placed between the prostate and rectal wall, thus providing a separation barrier. The SpaceOAR remains in place for about three months and is then absorbed and leaves the body in the patient's urine. This product is now available at essentially all proton centers and most IMRT centers as well.

Proton centers differ, somewhat, in the way they position the patient for treatment, but, as mentioned above, essentially all proton centers now offer the patient the space gel (SpaceOAR) option.

Advantages of Proton Treatment:

- Cure rates are comparable to surgery and radiation.
- No hospitalization is required; treatment is done on an outpatient basis.
- It is noninvasive; there is no pain, no blood loss, no trauma, and zero recuperation time.
- Incontinence from this procedure is practically unheard of. The reported statistic is significantly less than 1 percent.
- Because of the unique characteristic of the proton particle (Bragg Peak), the tumor area can be more precisely targeted and therefore there's less collateral damage and fewer side effects, including lower incidence of sexual dysfunction and impotence. A *WebMD Health News* article on Nov. 5, 2010 reported that in one study 18 months after treatment 94 percent of men remained sexually active following proton therapy.
- In addition to the prostate and capsule, a 5 to 12 mm margin around the gland and local seminal vesicles is also treated with protons, so any cancer in the margins is destroyed. This is significant for reasons discussed below.

Disadvantages of Proton Treatment:

- Requires eight weeks of treatment, five days a week. *This is changing dramatically with new, shorter hypofractionation protocols which will be explained later in this book. Very soon I expect the standard proton protocol to be four weeks or less.*

- Approximately 35 percent of the men treated report *some changes* in sexual potency. Patient surveys which I will cover later in this book, add important clarification to this.
- More expensive than other options and, while Medicare pays for this leading-edge treatment, many private insurers refuse to cover proton therapy, though this may be changing as well. (See Chapter 13 on The Medical Insurance Challenge)

One last point on proton treatment: All the statistics seem to point to the fact that proton treatment cure rates are *at least* as good as the "gold standard," surgery. When I was doing my due diligence, I found a comprehensive 10-year study published in the *International Journal of Radiation Oncology, Biology and Physics* (Vol. 59, No. 2, pp 348-352, 2004) that confirmed this. However, my research convinced me that I could expect even *better* results from proton therapy. Why? Because the routine procedure at Loma Linda University Cancer Center involved targeting the prostate, the capsule, the local seminal vesicles plus an extra 12-millimeter (half inch) margin, which is significant. This margin treats microscopic cancer cells that surgery might have missed. Further, the above studies were conducted on patients who received lower doses of proton radiation than is administered today. Recent dose escalation clinical trials have resulted in higher allowable proton radiation levels delivered to the tumor volume. One would expect cure rates to improve as more cancer-killing radiation finds its target. I'm convinced future studies will confirm this.

5. CRYOSURGERY

Cryosurgery – or cryoablation – involves the controlled freezing of the prostate gland in order to destroy the cancerous cells. Studies dating back to the 1960s showed this technique worked, but complications frequently arose due to the difficulty in precisely monitoring and controlling the freezing process. Modern techniques have reportedly improved delivery techniques and reduced complications.

Patients often go on a three- to six-month hormone therapy program to shrink the prostate prior to treatment.

Either general or spinal anesthesia is administered and then needle punctures are made in the perineum – the area between the anus and the scrotum. Cryo probes are then inserted to freeze the prostate to minus 40° Celsius. Multiple thermocouples or temperature-measuring devices are inserted to monitor the freezing process. A warming device is also inserted to protect the urethra. Two freezing cycles are performed, and a catheter is inserted to allow the bladder to be drained.

The procedure takes only a few hours and the patient is usually released the following day. The catheter must remain in place for about three weeks.

This technology is still developing and there isn't a large patient population from which to draw statistics. Overall, results have been mixed. Today, cryosurgery seems to be more popular as a salvage treatment when other treatments fail.

A study reported in the journal, *Urology* in March 2010 reported on a study involving 1,198 patients who had undergone whole prostate gland cryoablation at the Cleveland Clinic, MD Anderson Cancer Center, Columbia University, University of Calgary in Canada, and the International Society of Cryosurgery in Trieste, Italy. This study found that overall 77 percent of the patients were deemed to be cancer free five years after treatment. Specifically, 85 percent of the low-risk group were disease free; 73 percent of the intermediate-risk group were disease free; and 62 to 75 percent of the high-risk group were disease free at five years.

Advantages of Cryosurgery:

- Minimally invasive and minimal blood loss.
- Comparable cure rates to most other options.
- Low cost.
- Short treatment time, typically one day.
- Quick recovery/recuperation.
- Other traditional options are available if this treatment fails.

Disadvantages of Cryosurgery:

- Limited database; only a small number of patients have been treated.
- Impotence was reported in 91 percent of the cases according to the 2010 study reported in the journal, *Urology*, with only a small number of these regaining even partial potency.
- Incontinence rates are comparable to lower than the other options and seem to vary, depending on the practitioner administering the treatment.
- Other urinary system or rectal complications are possible.

6. HIFU – HIGH INTENSITY FOCUSED ULTRASOUND

HIFU (pronounced HIGH-foo) is a promising technology that heats tumors to near-boiling temperatures. HIFU has the potential to treat tumors of the prostate liver and lung without need for incision. And because it's minimally invasive, it has the potential for minimizing side effects, including impotence and incontinence, when used to treat prostate cancer.

There are two competing HIFU system manufacturers, Sonablate, made by Focus Surgery, and Albatherm, made by EDAP TMS, S.A.

In treating prostate cancer with HIFU, spinal or epidural anesthesia is administered, and a probe is placed in the rectum. The probe emits a beam of high intensity focused ultrasound, significantly increasing the temperature at the targeted volume. Different from radiotherapy, which "damages" DNA, programming cancerous cells to die-off, the intent of HIFU is to destroy the entire prostate.

The procedure takes from one to four hours and is typically done on an out-patient basis. Patients often arrive the day before treatment and travel home the day after the procedure. Follow-up can be handled by the patient's local urologist. A retropubic or Foley catheter must be worn for two to four weeks. Temporary urinary urgency and minor urinary discomfort are common after treatment.

HIFU can be repeated if the cancer returns and is still confined to the prostate. It's also growing in use as a salvage therapy when other prostate cancer treatments fail.

A five-year follow-up study at the University of Regensburg Germany was published in the journal, *Urology*. It was titled, "High-Intensity Focused Ultrasound for the Treatment of Localized Prostate Cancer: Five-year Experience." The article reported that 93 percent of the 137 men followed had negative biopsies five years later; 87 percent had constant PSA levels less than 1.0; and only two patients had PSA levels higher than 4.0.

John Rewcastle, PhD., Adjunct Assistant Professor of Radiology at the University of Calgary and medical director at Albatherm, believes that, "HIFU is the next frontier in prostate treatment."

Others have differing opinions: In an October 2008 article in *BottomLine Personal Magazine* titled "Prostate Cancer Breakthroughs – New Research is Saving Lives," Peter Scardino, M.D. (Memorial Sloan-Kettering Cancer Center) said, "There is not enough clinical data to show that HIFU is an effective way to treat prostate cancer. In fact, doctors in the U.S. are beginning to see recurrences in men treated with HIFU – men who might have been cured with proven therapy. Bottom line: New treatments for prostate cancer may be popular, but that doesn't mean they work."

In a 2008 *Johns Hopkins Health Alert*, H. Ballentine Carter, M.D., Professor of Urology, had two words of advice for men contemplating HIFU therapy for prostate cancer: "Buyer beware."

The New York Times ran an article in January 2008 that was somewhat negative on HIFU. And while citing some successes, they highlighted the cases of an Illinois executive who was treated with HIFU and was left impotent, incontinent, and with recurrent prostate cancer, and another individual whose cancer also returned.

Dr. Cary Robertson, a Duke urologist who has studied HIFU, reported that published research suggested that up to 50 percent of patients who undergo this therapy might lose all or part of their sexual function.

The FDA rejected approval of HIFU for treating prostate cancer according to *Harvard Medical School Health Publications* in 2014. An unpublished study at that time showed that HIFU wasn't highly effective. "Nearly one in three prostates treated with HIFU tested positive for cancer in biopsies taken two years after treatment. It also posed a high risk of side effects, with more than half of the men treated with high intensity focused ultrasound experiencing erectile dysfunction, urinary retention, incontinence or other health problems."

However, in early 2015, the FDA approved the first ultrasound system for the ablation of prostate tissue in the U.S., the Sonablate 450. Later that same year, the FDA approved the Ablatherm system.

In August 2018, the journal *European Urology* reported on a prospective study involving 625 men. HIFU was found to be an effective treatment for localized prostate cancer with high overall survival and high metastasis-free survival. Dr. Gerald Chodak reporting in *Medscape*, was somewhat critical of the study for three reasons: 1) 28 percent of the patients treated were low risk and could have easily done active surveillance and 55 percent were Gleason 3+4 and might have fallen into the same active surveillance category; 2) while the study showed a relatively high urinary continence rate, erectile dysfunction results were monitored, but not reported; and 3) the median follow-up was only 56 months, but a high percentage of the men were less than two years post-treatment and it's hard to draw meaningful conclusions with only two years of follow-up. Also, 25 percent of the patients treated had recurrences and were eligible to be re-treated.

I have communicated with nine former HIFU patients who were treated in Canada, the Dominican Republic, Mexico, and Australia. HIFU is also practiced in Europe, South America, Russia and Asia. Since the procedure is still relatively new, there's little data available.

The men I communicate with were all treated within the previous four years. Most indicated that, following treatment, their PSAs dropped quickly to very low levels. One reported non-detectable PSA, which is what you would expect if the prostate is "destroyed." Two were dealing with cancer recurrences – and one of them was having HIFU a second time for salvage. A fourth gentleman reported rising PSA, but a recurrence had not yet been confirmed.

Most reported some short-term incontinence, but all indicated their bladder control returned to normal after a few weeks.

One reported that he was impotent and had lost all sexual function. Three indicated there was reduced sexual function, and the rest said their sexual function had diminished, but was returning to normal. Like other treatments, ejaculate had mostly disappeared. Some were using ED medication to enhance sexual function.

Two reported incidents of urethral strictures from scar tissue beginning after treatment. One had to self-catheterize for a while in order to urinate. Out-patient medical procedures corrected the problem for both men. International HIFU reports that strictures occur with about 18 percent of the patients.

Overall, most were happy with their treatment decision, and said that if they had to make the decision again, they would choose HIFU.

Although data is limited and equipment and techniques are still changing, this treatment option shows promise.

Advantages of HIFU:

- Procedure can be done in one session.
- Minimally invasive (but not non-invasive).
- Rapid recovery.
- Potential to minimize side effects, especially urinary incontinence.
- HIFU can be repeated if the cancer returns and is still confined to the prostate.
- Medicare covers most of the HIFU cost in the U.S. But out-of-pocket expenses for treating uncovered physicians' and anesthesiologists' fees could be in the $9,000 to $12,000 range, according to HIFU Prostate Services.

Disadvantages of HIFU:

- Practitioner dependent. Results can vary by physician depending on level of experience.
- Patient must wear catheter for two to four weeks, occasionally longer.
- Potential risk from anesthesia.
- Potential for urethral strictures.
- Up to 50 percent of patients will lose all or part of their sexual function.

- If cancer has escaped the gland and is in the margins it would likely not be destroyed.
- Minimal data available on disease-free survival and side effects on which to draw conclusions or to make a choice with confidence.
- As of this writing – to my knowledge – HIFU is not covered by private (non-Medicare) insurers.

7. HORMONE ABLATION THERAPY OR ANDROGEN DEPRIVATION THERAPY

Hormone ablation therapy, or HAT, is also known as androgen deprivation therapy, ADT. The term, "ablation" means deprivation, and this therapy is all about shutting down the male sex hormones (androgens) which are known to feed prostate cancer. The predominant androgen in men is testosterone. Another term for this systemic therapy is "hormonal therapy."

Often the treatment involves the use of a combination of drugs such as Lupron, Casodex and Zoladex or their generic equivalent. These drugs typically prevent the testicles, which produce the testosterone, from getting the message to do so. Unpleasant as it sounds, hormone therapy is a form of "temporary chemical castration." A common side effect is loss of libido.

Depriving the cancer of testosterone does not kill cancer; it merely retards the growth of cancer cells. Studies have shown that over time, the cancer cells can learn to thrive without their source of testosterone. For this reason, some doctors prescribe "intermittent hormonal therapy." This treatment, as the term suggests, involves the cycling on and off of hormone therapy over differing periods of time, depending on such measurements as PSA and testosterone level. The intent here is to "hold down" the cancer while preventing the cancer cells from becoming "refractory," or resistant to hormone therapy.

Doctors have used hormone therapy for years to shrink prostates and large tumors prior to using other treatments for dealing with prostate cancer. They've also used hormone therapy in conjunction with other treatments (e.g. surgery or radiation), especially for moderate to advanced prostate cancers.

Some medical institutions have recently begun studies using hormone therapy alone for early- and mid-stage prostate cancers.

Surgical removal of the testicles (called orchiectomy or castration) is another way of shutting down production of testosterone. This procedure is occasionally performed on patients with advanced prostate cancer.

Advantages of Hormone Therapy:

- Noninvasive; no trauma; no blood loss; no hospitalization required.
- It can halt the growth of cancer while other options are being evaluated.
- Can be used as a "salvage" technique when other options fail.

Disadvantages of Hormone Therapy:

- Generally not considered a "cure," but a temporary measure to suppress cancer growth.
- Side effects can include some, or all of the following: Loss of sexual function, hot flashes, weight gain, breast enlargement, depression, fatigue, reduction in genital size, and reduction in muscle and bone mass. Most of these side effects are temporary, but can last many months after treatment, depending on how much time the patient was on hormonal therapy.

8. ACTIVE SURVEILLANCE

This used to be called "watchful waiting," and is not only a viable alternative to treatment, it's growing in popularity. The reason for this is that prostate cancer is often slow growing, and the patient might never experience any symptoms from slow-growing, indolent prostate cancer during his lifetime. Add to this the fact that all treatment options carry the possibility of life-altering side effects, and you can understand why active surveillance is an option that should be seriously considered.

Recently developed imaging technologies that can identify lesions for targeted biopsies as well as predict the aggressiveness of tumors also help doctors and patients decide on whether to consider active surveillance instead of aggressive treatment.

Active surveillance is not a "no treatment" decision, but rather a decision to treat if/when your cancer warrants treatment. A patient can choose to do active surveillance while monitoring PSA, having periodic DREs, doing periodic advanced imaging and follow-up biopsies as needed. If PSA progression or medical testing indicate disease progression beyond the indolent stage, then one of the several treatment options above could be considered.

Criteria for Active Surveillance

Active surveillance should be considered if the patient fits the following criteria:

- PSA below 10 and rising slowly
- Over 60 years of age
- Gleason score of 3+3=6 or possibly 3+4=7
- Only a small volume of cancer is found
- T-staging of T1c, i.e. no palpable tumor by DRE
- The cancer is confined to the prostate

Active surveillance is also a consideration for men with limited life expectancy or men with co-morbidities, i.e. other serious disorders or diseases (e.g. heart disease, very high blood pressure, poorly controlled diabetes), where doctors might feel it's in the patient's best interest to hold off on immediate therapy to avoid complications.

A healthy, 65-year-old man, with two of 12 biopsy cores showing cancer with a PSA of 5.4 and doubling time of four years, Gleason score 3+3 and staging T1c, would be an excellent candidate for active surveillance as his prostate cancer appears to be early stage and slow growing.

Older men with moderate-stage prostate cancer may also consider active surveillance, particularly if their PSA velocity is slow.

Each case is different, and each patient needs to be evaluated based on the above criteria and his life expectancy.

There are those who emotionally could not or would not consider active surveillance knowing there is cancer activity in their bodies. Even though they are candidates for active surveillance, they might take the risk of side effects from treatment if only to put their mind at ease that they have treated their cancer.

Typically, a patient who is on active surveillance would monitor PSA closely, perhaps every three months at first, shifting to every six months if PSA is relatively stable over time. In the past, a repeat biopsy, one or two years after the initial biopsy was often done to determine if there was any substantive change. In the absence of cancer growth and minimal PSA velocity, active surveillance may be continued indefinitely. With newer imaging technologies emerging, it's possible that periodic, follow-up invasive biopsies can be virtually eliminated when a patient is doing active surveillance.

A few years ago, *The New England Journal of Medicine* was recommending against active surveillance if life expectancy was greater than five years. With recent medical advances and newer imaging technologies, this is changing. More and more men are choosing active surveillance and are living long, normal lives. Also, research is under way to find ways for men with intermediate-stage prostate cancer to consider active surveillance.

One More Important Thing Men Do While on Active Surveillance

Much information has been developed over the past few years on the impact of diet and lifestyle on all forms of cancers as well as other deadly diseases.

- Stopping smoking
- Dietary changes
- Maintaining proper body weight
- Regular exercise

These important steps are beneficial no matter how healthy you are and no matter what health issue you're dealing with. They're especially beneficial to men who are practicing active surveillance.

I've learned much over the past 19 years about how these important steps can be critical factors in slowing, stopping and even reversing the growth of prostate cancer. Men doing active surveillance would be wise to pay close attention to these important steps to maintaining and improving health.

These topics will be covered in detail later in this book.

Advantages of Active Surveillance:

- Avoids the pain, trauma, potential blood loss, infection, complications from anesthesia, etc. which are all possible from the surgical option.
- Avoids the invasiveness of seeds and cryosurgery, and inconvenience and potential side effects from the various radiation options.
- Side effects from any of the major treatment options are virtually eliminated, therefore bladder control and sexual potency are maintained.

Disadvantages of Active Surveillance:

- Psychologically, the patient knows there is cancer growing in the prostate with no action being taken to destroy it. Some are uncomfortable living under these conditions.
- The cancer could conceivably grow unnoticed, spread beyond the prostate, limiting treatment options in the future.

Can men live with slow-growing cancer in their bodies? Absolutely. Keep in mind that a large percentage of men in their 80s and 90s have prostate cancer and don't know it. Autopsies on men who die in their 80s and 90s and older, often find cancer when the prostate is biopsied. There were never any symptoms; it never caused any harm; and it didn't need to be treated. The patient didn't know he had it and he died of something else. You are wise to keep active surveillance in mind when you're making your treatment decision.

An Important Milestone is Reached

I remember sitting in my home office, reflecting on all I had learned so far – from books, the Internet and my interviews. It struck me that I had reached an important milestone and fulfilled a promise I had made to myself two years earlier while standing next to my brother in the recovery room following his surgery.

That day, I promised myself, that if/when I was diagnosed with prostate cancer, I'd find an option that was less barbaric and intrusive than surgery, and one that would result in much less impact on my quality of life *after* treatment. I remember sitting in my office with my feet on the desk, a smug look on my face, and feeling great relief, realizing I had found *several* options that met these criteria.

I also remember wondering, "Why do so many men choose surgery, when just about all the other options afford them essentially the *same* chance of a cure, but without the trauma, blood loss, and side effects associated with surgery?" The answer, I would later discover, is that many men don't take the time to do their homework. They typically choose the specialty practiced by the physician who diagnosed them – their urologist.

I have no doubt most urologists believe their treatment is best. But so do the radiation oncologists, brachytherapists, cryotherapists, HIFU practitioners – and for that matter, watchful-waiting proponents, homeopaths, and alternative-medicine practitioners. So, it's up to the patient to do his due diligence and pick a treatment based on thorough analysis and a comprehensive evaluation of *all* the options. The treatment you choose may still fail to destroy/remove all the cancer, but at least you won't be second guessing yourself if you later learned there was another treatment option you would have chosen if you had known about it.

I truly had reached an important milestone. Surgery was off the table – pun intended.

CHAPTER 7

Proton Treatment is Beginning to Look More and More Attractive

"When you are patient enough to stop, look, listen, and asking what to do, you will always be shown how to do it."

– Lyanla Vanzant

Could This New Treatment Be for Me?

The more I read and heard about proton therapy, the more it felt like the right choice for me. The benefits: no trauma, no pain, no discomfort, minimal radiation damage to surrounding organs and tissue, and – minimal, if any, side effects. Most important, the statistical cure rates were at least comparable with those of the "gold standard," surgery, as well as the other major treatment methods.

But I still had some doubts and a lot of questions. This treatment procedure appeared to be relatively new. How many patients have been treated? How many had been cured? Are the claims of minimal side effects true? Is this procedure experimental? If so, would my insurance company pay for it?

Even if insurance paid for it, what about out-of-pocket cost for travel, car rental, and living expenses? And what about the inconvenience? The treatment would take eight weeks. In the fall of 2000, there was only one place in the world that offered this treatment – Loma Linda University Cancer Center in Southern California. I would have to relocate from Massachusetts to this unknown city for eight weeks, and possibly miss Thanksgiving and Christmas at home with my family.

And in the back of my mind was another burning question: *If this treatment is so good, why isn't it offered all over the world?*

The more I learned, it seemed, the more questions I had. And the more I learned about proton therapy, the more I *wanted* it to be right for me. But I had to be sure.

What is This "Loma Linda" Place?

I had never heard of Loma Linda before. So, I thought, what is this place that's offering this "unknown" treatment?

In my research, I learned that Loma Linda University Medical Center was established in 1905. It consists of eight health professional schools, six hospitals and more than 1,000 faculty physicians located in the Inland Empire of Southern California. The institution, I learned, is a global leader in education, research and clinical care, offering over 100 academic programs and healthcare to over 50,000 inpatients and 1.5 million outpatients every year. I would later learn that Loma Linda University Medical Center is where the "Baby Fae" baboon heart transplant took place in 1984, and where infant heart transplant surgery was pioneered. Loma Linda is a Seventh-day Adventist, faith-based health system with a mission "to continue the teaching and healing ministry of Jesus Christ." As a practicing Catholic, this last point resonated with me.

Questions for the Cancer Center

Nevertheless, I was getting anxious. I remember "beating myself up" one day and thinking, "It's been four weeks since my diagnosis, and all I've accomplished is to rule out surgery." But was I really being fair to myself? No. I had learned volumes about the other major treatment options, and I was zeroing in on one that could be right for me – one that still seemed too good to be true. It was time to learn more about proton therapy.

94

I called 1-800-PROTONS, the Loma Linda University Medical Center referral office. In contrast to my contacts with the other practitioners, the medical professionals at Loma Linda promptly returned my calls and always had time to talk with me. The people I spoke with at the Referral Office were extremely caring, professional, and responsive. I faxed them a list of questions – remember, this was almost 20 years ago – and the next day they faxed me the answers:

Q 1: Do you need to know the precise location of the tumor(s) for this therapy to be successful? In my case, my urologist tells me that the cancer sites are microscopic and can't be felt or seen by ultrasound.

A 1: *In terms of knowing the precise location of the tumor, we know from the biopsy that it's in your prostate gland, and, based on your cancer staging, in all probability it's confined there. Our radiation treatment field would include the entire gland, plus the capsule, the proximal (local) seminal vesicles, plus an extra 12-millimeter margin.*

Q 2: In my case, cancer was found only in the left lobe of my prostate. Would you treat *just* the left lobe, or the entire prostate? If you treat just the left lobe, how do you know there isn't cancer in the right lobe? The biopsy, after all is only a sample.

A 2: *As stated in the previous answer, the entire prostate gland is treated to give us the best chance of destroying all the cancer cells.*

Q 3: How do you protect my urethra, which runs through the middle of my prostate?

A 3: *You are quite right; the urethra runs through the prostate and thus is in the radiation path. However, the urethra is surprisingly tolerant of radiation and it typically handles the radiation well. Occasionally there are temporary side effects such as burning during urination, and possibly spasms of the urethra. We have medications that can treat these symptoms, which typically subside after the treatment ends.*

Q 4: I read that proton therapy is suited for "localized, solid tumors." Does this mean it's not suited for my early-stage prostate cancer, which is microscopic and cannot be seen by ultrasound?

A-4: *No. Proton therapy is highly suited for early-stage prostate cancer such as yours. We have a well-defined target – the prostate gland – even though we cannot see the cancer cells themselves.*

Q 5: How many prostate cancer patients have been treated at Loma Linda? What are the statistics on cure rate, especially ranked by pretreatment PSA and Gleason score? Can you send me a copy of the statistics?

A 5: *We have treated hundreds of prostate cancer patients. I have mailed you published information on the statistics you requested.*

Q 6: Before I travel to California, I'd like to speak with prostate cancer patients who've received treatment there. Can you give me some names and telephone numbers?

A 6: *Yes, I will fax you a list of prior patients who are on a volunteer call list and are willing to speak with you.*

Q 7: What are the typical side effects of this treatment? What would you expect in my case?

A 7: *Side effects can include fatigue, urinary problems, impotence, possible increase in frequency of stools, rectal irritation and/or discomfort. The severity of these varies from person to person and depends on your health, present urinary symptoms (which I see in your case is none), and energy level going into treatment. Generally, most patients tolerate this treatment very well and report minimal side effects.*

Q 8: It appears that proton therapy is only *sometimes* effective in killing cancer cells. See the following quotes. Am I misinterpreting these statements from Internet publications?

"While both normal and cancerous cells go through this repair process (after proton therapy treatment), a cancer cell's ability to repair itself is *frequently* inferior - - -"

"Damaging the DNA destroys specific cell functions, which *may* include the ability to divide or proliferate - - -"

"A cancer cell's ability to repair molecular injury is *frequently* inferior. As a result, cancer cells sustain *more permanent* damage and subsequent cell death than occurs in the normal cell population."

A 8: *I think if you are interpreting these statements as being unique to proton beam treatment and its efficacy, then yes, that's probably a misinterpretation. No cancer therapy is guaranteed to be 100 percent effective, unfortunately. That's also true for surgery, all forms of radiation, chemotherapy, etc. The sentences you quote refer to cancer cells in general, and so they use words like "frequently," "may," etc. Almost any cell in the body can lose its ability to regulate its growth normally and become cancerous, and as they start out as different kinds of cells (i.e. lung cells, glandular cells, brain cells, etc.) they don't all behave exactly the same way. This in turn means that they can respond to treatments differently. Some respond to chemotherapy very well, some do not. Some respond better to radiation than others. We know that the proton beam can kill cancer in the prostate. But we can never be absolutely sure that none of those cells has escaped and traveled to another part of the body. As compared to other forms of cancer that are considered aggressive and metastasize readily, prostate cancer is relatively slow growing.*

Q 9: Is my specific case a good fit for proton therapy?

A 9: *Yes, your cancer is considered early stage. Early stage cancers typically have the best outcomes.*

Q 10: Is surgery no longer an option if proton therapy fails?

A 10: *Many urologists will not do surgery on someone who has had radiation therapy for prostate cancer, but some specialists* can and will do this procedure. But when radiation therapy fails, it usually fails because the cancer had previously moved outside the field that was treated. If this is the case, why consider surgery to remove the gland? There are other aspects of this issue that would best be discussed with your doctor if you come in for a consult.

Q 11: How much total time should I expect to spend at Loma Linda including pre-testing and preparations?

A 11: *The treatment is eight weeks in duration – Monday through Friday, daily treatments. A CT scan of your pelvis will be done to be used to plan your treatment and it takes one to two weeks to start treatment once that CT is done.*

Q 12: Can you tell me about living arrangements and costs?

A 12: *There are numerous options available to you. I will send you this information in the mail.*

Q 13: Based on what you've seen of my specific case and considering all the treatment options available to me, what treatment option would you select if you were in my shoes?

A 13: *That decision is, of course, up to you. Even though I'm not a man, I think I can understand not wanting to have to live with some of the possible side effects of prostate cancer treatment. Proton therapy is as effective as surgery or conventional radiation and with generally fewer side effects.*

Q 14: In my case, what is the degree of urgency for treatment? (ASAP, this month, this year, next year?)

A 14: *This is hard to answer and best discussed with a physician. I would say that if you get treatment in a couple of months it should be fine. I think waiting a year may not be a wise thing to do.*

Q 15: If I qualify, when could you take me?

A 15: *We could schedule you for a consult in about a month.*

I was satisfied with these answers, and within a few days I would have new ammunition. I would have data, which compared proton therapy with other treatment options. I was elated by their promise to send me the names of men who had received proton treatment. Talking with them, I knew, would be a major factor in making my decision.

As promised, the next day I received a fax with a list of 30 names, addresses, treatment dates, and phone numbers. This astounded me! For a month I had been struggling to get the names of men who had received various forms of treatment such as surgery, EBRT, brachytherapy, and cryo, and was met with formidable resistance. The response from the doctor's office was typically, "We need to respect the privacy of the patient and cannot give out names" (This was before today's strict HIPAA regulations on patient confidentiality). I told them I didn't want to invade their privacy. I just wanted to talk with them about their experience of treatment, and they could do that anonymously, "Give them my number, have them call me," I pleaded. I had questions only someone on the "receiving end" of the treatment could answer.

The doctors and their nurses representing the other treatment options seemed "put off" by my request. They told me *they* could answer all my questions, and there really wasn't any need for me to talk with their patients. The more they resisted, the more I persisted.

I have always believed that a *salesman* will tell you almost anything to make the sale. It's the *customer* who will give you the *real* story about a product or service. He/she has nothing to gain or lose by being totally honest. In all my business dealings, I had relied heavily on customer satisfaction when choosing a vendor for a product or service. I also relied heavily on reference checks when hiring key people to work for me – just one more way of checking with a former "customer."

When I received the list of former proton patients, I established a plan. I would call every man on the list, beginning with those who were treated in the early 1990s. I prepared a list of questions, and typed up a survey sheet where I would collect 22 pieces of data on every man I spoke with (remember, I'm a "recovering engineer!"). I planned to ask each his age, cancer stage (PSA, Gleason score, T-score), when they were treated, short and long-term side effects, and much more.

Then the thought occurred to me, "How do I know these folks from Loma Linda didn't 'stack the deck?' Maybe they sent me a list of their success cases. How could I be sure I would be speaking with a representative group of former patients?" The solution to this dilemma was simple. As part of my survey, I would ask each man to give me the names of two patients he met while in treatment. If they spent eight weeks in that small town, surely, they would have developed relationships with other proton patients.

I remember sleeping well that night, knowing that I was about to add much to my knowledge base in the coming days.

My Survey

Following is the survey form I used for my interviews with former proton patients.

Name: _____ Phone: _____ Date: _____

Age when treated? _____ Current Age: _____ Treatment End Date: _____

Cancer Stage (T1, T2, etc.): ___ Palpable Tumor by DRE? ___Gleason Score: _____

Name of Insurance Company: _____ Did they pay? _____

Any side effects (short term, long term)?_____
_____

Current condition (PSA, symptoms)?_____
_____

Any other form of treatment done, such as hormone, photon (x-ray) radiation or surgery?_____
_____

What major factors influenced your decision to choose Proton? _____
_____
_____

What was your experience of Loma Linda and proton treatment?_____
_____
_____

What was your urologist's reaction to your decision to choose Proton? _____
_____

Who was your doctor and case manager? Would you recommend them? _____
_____

Would you make the same decision again? _____

What other information can you give me to help me with my decision? _____
_____

Can you give me the names and phone numbers of two men you know who went through Proton treatment?_____
_____
_____

Survey Results

I was pleasantly surprised by the receptivity of the men I called, as well as their friendliness and willingness to share intimate details of their diagnosis, treatment and follow-up. I would later learn that men with prostate cancer feel a bonding, or sense of brotherhood, and generally go out of their way to help others facing the same challenges.

Some of the men on the list had moved or changed phone numbers and were unreachable, but I was able to contact 20. Each happily answered all my questions, and freely provided the names of others with whom they were treated. Over a six-day period I spoke with 56 former proton patients. And I had certainly bracketed my areas of interest: ages 51 to 84, PSAs 2.5 to 27, Gleason scores 4 to 9, stages T1c to T3 (A to C).

What did I learn from these interviews? Volumes! I had struck gold! Following is a summary of what I heard from these former proton patients:

Side Effects

Most claimed that the side effects were minimal to non-existent. Eight men (14 percent) reported some occasional, minor rectal bleeding, which began several months after treatment ended. In six of the eight cases it had stopped. The other two reported it was minimal and they expected it to go away. I later learned that temporary, minor rectal bleeding is not uncommon with radiation treatment. It's a result of a phenomenon called radiation-induced neovascularization. Healthy cells on the interior wall of the rectum that were exposed to some radiation – because of the 12 mm margin treated – typically repair themselves, forming new blood vessels. Occasionally these blood vessels "leak" blood into the stool. This condition is usually temporary, painless, and it almost always goes away on its own.

A few of those I spoke with reported some urinary urgency or urinary burning during the later stages of treatment, which subsided after treatment ended.

Most reported normal sex lives, albeit with significantly less ejaculate (all treatment options reduce or eliminate ejaculate, usually with no impact on sexual performance or pleasure).

Those with more advanced cancers who were on adjunct hormone therapy were experiencing a loss of libido, which they said they "hoped" was temporary. One gentleman who had stopped hormone therapy admitted to not regaining sexual function. Twelve

(21 percent) felt their sexual potency had diminished somewhat following proton treatment. When questioned further, the common theme was more difficulty achieving erections, and/or less firmness with erections. One respondent offered that, "Sex has definitely changed for me. I'm down to only twice a week! But my age might have something to do with it. I was 84 last month."

Most of those with diminished potency who tried erectile dysfunction medications reported positive results.

None of the 56 reported having any problems with incontinence. Let me repeat that: *Not a single person reported having any problems with bladder control or urine leakage.* This was my *number one* concern.

I was feeling a lot better about proton treatment.

Current PSA

Every person I spoke with felt he was in a much better space for having chosen proton treatment. PSAs were dramatically reduced in every case. All but one reported PSAs below 1.0. Those treated three or more years earlier felt they had reached their PSA nadir (low point). Several indicated their PSAs were "still coming down."

Other Treatments They Received

About a third of the men I spoke with were given some additional form of treatment – photon radiation and/or hormone therapy. Photon radiation was prescribed, in addition to proton therapy, for those whose cancers might have progressed beyond the prostate gland as indicated by DRE, high PSA, and/or high Gleason score. Photon radiation is used to treat the entire prostate bed including lymph nodes. Typically, the same total amount of radiation is delivered, but it's split between the two forms.

Hormone treatment in conjunction with proton or proton/photon was common for men with very large prostates and/or advanced cancers.

Temporary side effects from hormones included hot flashes, loss of sexual desire, and occasionally enlarged breasts. Photon radiation occasionally resulted in temporary fatigue. Other than fatigue, those who were treated with proton and photon didn't seem to experience any more severe side effects than those treated with proton alone.

Major Factors Influencing Their Decision

Surprisingly, a large percentage of the men I spoke with were scientists, engineers, physicists, doctors, lawyers, educators, and business leaders. They all seemed to have analytical minds, and an interest and ability to review, digest, and understand technical information.

They all did their homework and researched the alternatives. None blindly accepted their urologist's initial recommendation, which in almost every case was surgery. All were convinced that radiation kills cancer; that proton therapy is the most advanced and precise form of radiation therapy; that their chance of a cure with proton therapy was at least as good as other standard treatments; and that side effects with protons were minimal, giving them the best chance of a high quality of life after treatment.

Their Experience of Loma Linda And the Treatment Process

If there were any doubts in their minds as to the efficacy of the treatment or the medical professionals at the hospital, they were quickly dispelled when they visited the proton treatment facility at the Loma Linda University Cancer Center and met with the staff. Every respondent expressed superlatives about the doctors, case managers, technicians, and support staff. It sounded too good to be true.

Urologists' Reaction

Most of the men I spoke with told me their urologists were opposed to their choice of proton treatment. Their doctors described the treatment as "experimental, investigational, early stage, unproven, or dangerous." Some urologists told their patients to "find yourself another doctor if you choose proton treatment." A few were more open minded and offered their best wishes. Only one urologist indicated he knew of proton therapy, that it was a viable alternative, and he supported the decision.

Doctor and Case Manager

In late 2000 there were several radiation oncologists at Loma Linda. Lucky for me, I gained knowledge on all of them because of the large number of patients I spoke with. And the responses made me smile. Each patient felt he had the best doctor at the institution and strongly suggested that I choose his doctor. Not one respondent said anything negative about his radiation oncologist. Bottom line: All the physicians there were superb according to my survey, and they were highly respected by their patients.

I later learned something else about proton therapy that sets it apart from surgery and brachytherapy. *Proton therapy is not particularly practitioner dependent.* It really didn't matter which doctor I chose. The procedures are all documented and well established. And following the initial CT scan, the customized treatment protocol is reviewed by a team of physicians, dosimetrists and physicists; i.e. every single case is reviewed by a *team* of competent professionals.

Cancer Recurrence

One of the men I interviewed reported his cancer had returned. It's interesting to note that he was on the original call list I received from Loma Linda, not one I'd found through my survey. He reported that his PSA began to rise three years after treatment ended, and that a biopsy of his prostate detected no cancer. He said that prior to treatment his cancer had moved outside the area treated and the proton therapy did its job killing the cancer in his prostate. He told me the quality of his life hadn't changed one bit since he was treated; he had no regrets for having chosen proton therapy; and he highly recommended it to me. He was in the process of researching salvage treatment options and was optimistic about his future.

Would You Make the Same Decision Again?

This question received an unequivocal and resounding *yes* from every respondent.

But What About Andy Grove?

This all seemed too good to be true. But something was still troubling me. If proton therapy is this good, then why didn't Andy Grove choose it when he was treated in the mid-90s? He was a wealthy business leader who could have had any treatment at any medical institution in the world. Why didn't he choose proton therapy? I speculated that it was because he was a busy executive and couldn't afford to be away from his office for eight weeks.

To answer this question, I sent him one last email and asked, "Mr. Grove, I've been researching treatment options, and I am leaning toward proton beam therapy at Loma Linda University Cancer Center. In your position, you could have chosen any treatment, anywhere in the world. Proton therapy appears to me to be the best option available by a wide margin. Why didn't you choose it?"

His answer was right to the point, "Bob, I had never heard of proton beam therapy, so it was never a treatment I considered."

To my knowledge Andy Grove lived the rest of his life free of prostate cancer. "The father of Silicon Valley" passed away in 2016 at the age of 79. Though he was known to have suffered from Parkinson's disease for years, the cause of his death was not reported.

I will always be grateful to this extraordinary man for taking time from his busy schedule on several occasions to help a frightened 57-year-old prostate cancer victim who was starving for information and struggling with his treatment decision. I also learned a lesson about the importance and the value of helping others and paying it forward. I didn't know this at the time, but I would soon be devoting the bulk of my life to this mission.

CHAPTER 8

My Treatment Decision

"Two roads diverged in a wood, and I took the one less traveled by, and that has made all the difference."

– Robert Frost

The Value of Talking with Other Men

Looking back at all my efforts in researching the alternatives, clearly the greatest value for me was in speaking with men who had chosen each of the treatment options. They filled in all the missing pieces, most of which I would never have found on the Internet or in the countless books and articles that have been written on prostate cancer.

Tip: Before making your treatment choice, speak with several (preferably 10 or more) men who have had each form of treatment you are considering. Their personal experience will be invaluable to you in making the decision that is best for you.

The Process of Elimination

I was clearly leaning toward proton therapy, but I had to be sure. Sometimes it pays to be an anal-retentive, obsessive-compulsive, recovering engineer.

I quickly ruled out active surveillance. I felt I was too young and had too many years for the cancer to grow and metastasize, and my PSA had been rising somewhat rapidly during the previous two years. Why should I give this thing growing inside me a chance to migrate beyond the gland and move into my lymph nodes, eventually metastasizing and traveling to the rest of my body? No – active surveillance was not for me.

Cryoablation was relatively new, and there were minimal statistics on which to base a decision. I also had difficulty finding people to talk with who had received this treatment. And, what little I had heard about side effects, particularly urinary incontinence, frightened me.

I couldn't think of one valid reason for keeping radical prostatectomy on the "short list." It's major surgery; it's a complex and bloody procedure; the side effects are many and are more severe than the alternatives; results are extremely practitioner dependent; and 0.5 percent of the patients my age die on the operating table. It works only if the cancer is totally confined to the prostate, whereas most of the other treatments provide the added benefit of treating a certain "margin" around the prostate. Surgery was definitely off the list, and when I admitted this, I felt a huge weight lifted off my shoulders.

Laparoscopic radical prostatectomy was brand new in 2000, and I couldn't find any published information on the subject. I've since learned that, while patients recover more quickly from this type of surgery, the complications and side effects are essentially the same as with open surgery, and sometimes worse. So, it too was off my list.

This left brachytherapy, 3D-conformal external beam radiation therapy, IMRT, and proton treatment.

I continued to search the Internet, seek out new books, and interview former patients. Facts began to emerge that shed some new light on brachytherapy. Nineteen percent of the seeds implanted in the prostate tend to dislodge and migrate to different parts of the body. Some pass through the urethra and leave the body with the urine; others find their way to the lungs. I learned that the half-life of the radiation in these seeds was very short. Nevertheless, the thought of having even low-level radioactive seeds settling in my lungs was disconcerting.

I continued my interviews with former patients representing the remaining treatment options and learned of two cases of incontinence connected with seed implants. One attorney who had chosen seeds, told me he carried two briefcases – one with his legal material and the other full of diapers. He said he couldn't sit through a meeting longer than one hour without having to change his diaper. This bothered me even more than the issue of seed migration.

108

There also appeared to be a higher incidence of bladder-neck stricture and urinary-tract blockage with seeds. I assumed that was due to the significantly higher dose of radiation to the urethra, which passes through the center of the prostate.

Earlier I mentioned that success with brachytherapy was extremely practitioner dependent. I was learning that in addition to killing the cancer, treatment success is also measured in terms of factors such as seed migration.

The few "premier" brachytherapy specialists were practically untouchable. I attempted to make an appointment with one and was told it would be several months before I could see him. Even then I might find he wouldn't take me as a patient, or I might be "diverted" to one of his associates.

For all the above reasons, I took brachytherapy off the list, and decided I would reconsider seeds, only if I could have the procedure done by Dr. John Blasko at the Seattle Prostate Institute.

The more I investigated 3D-CRT, the more I was discovering its use to be in conjunction with other treatments such as surgery, hormones, or proton. It seemed that conformal photon (X-ray) radiation, with its broad range, "shotgun" or "carpet-bomb" delivery of radiation was good for "mopping up" around the tumor site, especially if the cancer was more advanced and there was a high probability it had escaped the gland. But I was convinced this option carried with it a much higher probability of undesirable side effects.

IMRT made a lot of sense and really had my interest, but I saw two negatives. First, in 2000 it was still relatively new. There was practically no data available on this option, and I was having great difficulty finding former IMRT patients to interview. And second, IMRT still used photon (X-ray) radiation, and that meant a higher probability of collateral damage – side effects.

Proton treatment was looking better and better.

Nick DeWolf and His Decision Matrix

There's something about prostate cancer that makes a fraternity from its victims. Once I broke through the resistance of the doctors, I found patients were much more than willing to share information. All along the way, I met countless former patients who gave generously of their time to tell me their story and help me in my decision-making process. None was more helpful than Nick DeWolf.

Nick was diagnosed in 1996 and received a combination proton/photon treatment at Loma Linda. Before making his decision, he did exhaustive research into the alternatives and examined each technology in detail. As co-founder of Teradyne and now a retired "technocrat," Nick was comfortable wallowing in such terms as atoms, protons, photons, rads, cobalt-gray, ionization, and apoptosis.

As a service to his fellow man, Nick developed a comprehensive website where he methodically chronicled his journey.

I discovered Nick's website one Sunday afternoon while surfing the Internet and I read everything he wrote, explored every link and studied every chart and graph. One thing caught my attention: his "Decision Matrix."

Nick prepared his own somewhat subjective analysis of the four options he was considering: Proton, EBRT, surgery, and surgery plus X-ray. He identified all the factors he considered in his decision-making process, which included such things as probability of a cure, convenience, and short- and long-term side effects. Some factors were rated based on probabilities of occurrence; other factors were given weighted values, and then scored based on his research.

With Nick's permission, I have reproduced his decision matrix here along with his introduction:

Here is a matrix that may assist you in making your treatment choice. Each factor was weighted by its maximum (subjective importance) and my judgment (subjective) of my odds. Bigger values mean worse results. Other patients would alter the values widely, but this reasoning made my choice very easy.

		Radiation		Surgery	
		Proton	**X-ray**		
Include X-ray phase 2?	-	Yes	Yes	No	Yes
Hormone Adjuvant (months)		No	3	4-6	4-6
Days away from home	-	60	60	8	70
Days to ¾ recovery		0	0	80	80
Cost (relative)		30	15	15	25
Scoring	**Max**	G u e s t i m a t i o n s			
Likelihood of recurrence	500	50	100	200	50
Likelihood of induced cancer	100	5	10	0	10
Operating room traumas	100	0	0	50	50
Subtotal points:	**700**	**55**	**110**	**250**	**110**
Short term side effects					
Pain	50	0	0	20	20
Incontinence	15	0	5	15	15
Frequency of urination	15	5	10	15	15
Diarrhea	15	5	10	10	15
Exhaustion	40	10	10	20	25
Loss of Sexual Pleasure	25	5	5	15	15
Erectile Impotence	15	4	8	10	15
Inconvenience	25	10	10	5	12
Subtotal:	**200**	**39**	**58**	**110**	**132**
Longer term side effects					
Rectal & bladder damage	100	6	12	10	20
Pain	250	0	4	60	60
Incontinence	100	4	8	20	25
Frequency of urination	50	4	6	15	20
Diarrhea	100	4	6	10	15
Exhaustion	200	5	6	50	50
Loss of sexual pleasure	150	10	15	80	80
Erectile impotence	40	4	8	20	20
Infertility	10	3	3	10	10
Inconvenience	100	5	5	20	30
Subtotal	**1100**	**45**	**73**	**290**	**325**
Grand Total	**2000**	**139**	**241**	**650**	**567**
	Worst	*Proton*	*X-ray*	*Surgery*	

111

This approach really resonated with me. It was 9 p.m. when I finished exploring Nick's site. Since he kindly provided a link with his email address and an offer to respond to questions, I sent him an email with my phone number and asked if I could talk with him.

An hour later, at 10 p.m., my phone rang. It was Nick DeWolf. We spoke for two hours. I was impressed with his intellect and his candor. He graciously answered all my questions and offered to make himself available at any time if I had more questions or just wanted to talk. I remember hanging up the phone that night making a promise that if I beat this disease, I would do everything I could to help newly diagnosed men the way Nick DeWolf helped me.

Time to Visit Loma Linda

Although I was about 90 percent sure I wanted to do proton therapy, I hadn't made up my mind. What was it going to take? What would convince me that proton treatment was the best option? After wrestling with these questions for a while, the answer became obvious. I had to see, feel and touch proton therapy. I had to visit the facility, look at the equipment, and speak with the people who practiced this technology.

During the dozens of hours of patient interviews, I came across two gentlemen who had made their mark at Loma Linda. They had endeared themselves with doctors and staff with their charm, their humor, and the dozens of boxes of doughnuts they took to the proton treatment center each morning for the radiation therapists.

Both were on the patient call list the hospital had sent me. So, I called Joe Gazzola and Joe Praught, and asked for an introduction to the radiation oncologist who treated them, Dr. Carl Rossi. The "two Joes" told me that the way to reach Dr. Rossi was through his nurse/case manager, an extraordinary lady named Sharon Hoyle. I would later give her the pseudonym, "Florence Nightingale."

I called Sharon, introduced myself as a friend of "the two Joes," and asked for her assistance in seeing Dr. Rossi. Sharon arranged the appointment and offered one other suggestion: As long as I was making the trip across country, why not plan to have my CT scan and custom immobilization pod fabricated on the same visit? This would save me two to four weeks and another cross-country trip if I decided to choose the treatment (she knew I would). If I decided *not* to do the treatment, I would have to pay for these things out of pocket. I agreed.

I flew to Ontario airport in California, rented a car, and stayed at a local motel that offered discounts to Loma Linda patients. The next morning, I drove to the medical center and was instantly impressed by its size. The San Bernardino Valley sits between two mountain ranges, and most of the land in the valley is flat. Houses and commercial buildings are generally one to three stories. Towering above everything else in the valley was the Loma Linda University Medical Center (LLUMC).

The medical center buildings were white and surrounded by white support buildings, student and staff dormitories, and a chapel. The grounds and parking areas were meticulously maintained. Despite the desert climate, the grounds were lush with green grass and flowers. A helicopter was landing on the roof of the main building as I searched for a parking space in one of their huge parking lots. I later learned that LLUMC is a major trauma center for Southern California and that medivac helicopters routinely shuttle patients in from hundreds of miles away.

First Impressions

High on a tower over the main entrance of the hospital was a large cross and the words, "Loma Linda University Medical Center A Seventh-day Adventist Institution." I didn't consider myself an overly religious person at the time, but seeing the cross and reading those words gave me an immediate feeling of peace and comfort.

A security officer smiled and greeted me as I approached the front door. I was warmly welcomed by the receptionist at the main desk, given a visitor's pass, and directed to the proton treatment reception desk.

To my surprise, the proton center was three stories beneath the ground and directly under the children's hospital. I later learned that for safety reasons, construction was done beneath the earth, and the critical systems were surrounded by 14-foot-thick concrete-and-steel walls.

Sharon Hoyle was there to welcome me, take down some information, put me completely at ease, and usher me into Dr. Rossi's office.

I gave Dr. Rossi my paperwork, which included my medical history and pathology reports; and we discussed my case in great detail. He answered all my questions clearly, concisely, and honestly. I was impressed with his knowledge, his intellect, his manner, his humility, and the amount of uninterrupted time he gave me. I later learned that this is the norm at the institution. Patients aren't just numbers; they are "guests," and their visitor's badge identifies them as such.

Orientation Tour

Next, I was introduced to Gerry Troy, a social worker who was head of patient services for the proton center. Gerry led a two-hour tour of the facility, explaining the systems and technology. I remember thinking, "How can a "shrink" be this knowledgeable about the sophisticated technology of proton therapy?" "Gerry-the-Shrink" would later become a good friend.

Gerry explained in detail how the proton particle was extracted from hydrogen gas, introduced to the system, sped-up in a particle accelerator – called a synchrotron – and delivered to the treatment rooms. He also explained how the prostate was imaged three dimensionally by the CT scan; how the dosimetrists, physicists and radiation oncologists custom tailor a treatment plan for each patient; and how focusing devices, called apertures and boluses were constructed for each patient in order to conform the proton beam precisely to the target area.

He also showed us where and how the immobilization pod was made to ensure each patient is placed in precisely the same position every day for treatment. And, he explained how a small water-filled balloon was used to protect the rectum during the daily treatments. This last point certainly caught my attention.

Gerry then took us three floors down to the treatment areas. There I saw three giant gantries and a "fixed-beam" treatment room. Each gantry was three stories high, consisting of more than 100 tons of steel and concrete, and designed to rotate within extremely tight tolerances around the patient being treated.

A few days earlier, I wasn't sure what to expect as I conjured up images from my home in Massachusetts. But what I saw was nothing like what I expected. This was not some "fly-by-night" Frankenstein laboratory, with mad scientists scurrying about. What I saw was a Star-Wars-type, modern, super-clean facility, staffed by competent professionals.

That evening, at the suggestion of "the two Joes," I attended one of the weekly Wednesday night support group meetings. This popular meeting was attended by prospective patients (like me), current patients, former patients, and others. New patients, called "newbies," share stories of how they discovered proton therapy. Patients who are completing treatment, called "graduates," talk about their eight-week odyssey, usually in humorous terms, often accompanied by poetry, music, or comedy skits. Visiting graduates, called "alumni," often return to report how they're doing months or years after treatment.

The meeting was scheduled to begin at 5:30 p.m. I arrived at 5:15 p.m. and thought I was in the wrong place. The hallway outside the meeting room was jammed with high-spirited people who were lined up for sandwiches, cookies, and fruit drinks. Most of the chairs in the meeting room were occupied, and the remaining ones were disappearing fast. Everyone was smiling; some were laughing; and the atmosphere was festive. It felt like I had walked in on a group of people who had won the lottery – and in a way I had.

Gerry Troy called the meeting to order. It took two or three minutes to quiet the crowd and then Gerry began to talk. Without any introduction, he said:

A man from Texas, driving a Volkswagen Beetle, pulls up next to a guy in a Rolls Royce at a stop sign. Their windows are open, and he yells at the guy in the Rolls, "Hey, you got a telephone in that Rolls?"

The guy in the Rolls replies: "Yes, of course I do."
"I got one too… see?" the Texan says.
"Uh, yes that's very nice."
"You got a fax machine too?" the Texan asks.
"Why, actually, yes I do."
"I do too! See, it's right here," brags the Texan.

The light is about to turn green and the man in the Beetle says: "So, do you have a double bed in the back there?"

"NO! Do you?"

"Yep, got my double bed right in the back," the Texan replies. The light turns and the Beetle takes off.

Well, the guy in the Rolls is not about to be one-upped, so he immediately goes to a customizing shop and orders them to put in a double bed on the back of the Rolls. About two weeks later, the job is finally done.

He picks up his car and drives all over town looking for the Volkswagen Beetle with the Texas plates. Finally, he finds it parked alongside the road, so he pulls his Rolls up next to it.

The windows on the Volkswagen are all fogged up and he feels somewhat awkward about it, but he gets out of his newly modified Rolls and taps on the foggy window of the Volkswagen.

The man in the Volkswagen finally opens a window and peeks out. The guy in the Rolls says, "Hey, remember me?"

"Yeah, I remember you," says the Texan. "What's up?"

"Check this out… I got a double bed installed in my Rolls."

The Texan in the Volkswagen exclaims: "YOU GOT ME OUT OF THE SHOWER TO TELL ME THAT?"

The room erupted in laughter. Then someone from the back of the room raised his hand and said, "I've got one better than that," and he proceeded to tell *his* joke. After two or three more, Gerry started to make his announcements. He ran down the list of upcoming activities including such things as, "*The Movers and Shakers* group will meet on Thursday evening; the *Lunch Bunch* is going to *The Little Fisherman* restaurant on Friday; *Pod Partners* will meet on Monday at 3:30 p.m.; this week's restaurant tour will be at the Elks Lodge; we have some free tickets for the *San Bernardino Symphony Orchestra* concert next week; the extended proton tour will be held at 10:00 a.m.

116

on Saturday; tickets for the *Getty Museum* tour will be available on Friday, etc. The announcements went on for almost 10 minutes.

Next, Gerry asked if there were any "graduates" in the audience. Nine people raised their hands. Gerry called on them one by one, and each gave a "graduation speech." The speeches included poems, songs, and humorous accounts of each patient's experience at Loma Linda. They had us laughing one minute and crying the next. All expressed their sincere appreciation to the staff for their extraordinary experience.

The fun continued. Next Gerry asked if there were any "alumni" present. One by one, the former patients stood up, and recounted their journey through and since treatment. Alumni ranged from one man who had been treated for prostate cancer six years earlier and was doing "great," to a young woman who was successfully treated for an inoperable brain tumor a year before. All were in good spirits and thanked and praised LLUCC and the Lord for the "gift" they had been given. The spiritual atmosphere was evident in this room, which was full of laughter, tears and camaraderie that Wednesday evening.

Finally, Gerry asked for the "newbies" to identify themselves. About 15 hands went up. Most were prostate cancer patients from the U.S., Europe and Australia. They reported their pretreatment PSAs and Gleason scores and spoke about how they learned about proton treatment. None seemed fearful or anxious about the treatment they were just beginning. Was I the only one in the room worried about this dreaded disease and proton therapy?

I looked at my watch; it was almost 8 p.m. Where had the past 2 ½ hours gone? Why is everyone so cheery? The whole experience was beginning to feel surreal. "This room is filled with cancer patients," I thought, "How can they be so happy?"

I later learned that this meeting was just one of several psychosocial programs that LLUCC has instituted as part of its *Make Man Whole* mission.

Decision Made

While walking through the beautiful grounds of the Loma Linda University Cancer Center the next day, and reflecting on the events since my arrival – the cross on the tower, the warm reception, the meeting with Dr. Rossi and Sharon Hoyle, the tour of the proton treatment center, and the Wednesday night meeting – I made my decision. It was proton treatment for me!

I told Sharon Hoyle, my case manager, about my decision. She congratulated me and directed me to the team of people who would build my immobilization pod and do the CT scan.

The Pod, the Scan and My First Balloon

The immobilization pod is an approximately 7-foot-long, half-tube, completely open, and constructed of PVC. I was asked to put on a one-size-fits-none hospital gown, often called a "johnny." This cover-up is often the butt of jokes – no pun intended – because of the embarrassment it causes patients. It's a short gown, tied in the back, often leaving one's backside exposed.

I donned the johnny and climbed into the pod, which was lined with a soft fabric. It felt a little like climbing into a coffin.

Then they gave me my first balloon. I can't say it was uncomfortable. I learned this device is an infant enema wand, a piece of hollow, semi-rigid rubber, the diameter of a pencil, about five inches long, with what appeared to be a condom stretched over it. The technician coated it with KY Jelly and inserted it in my rectum. Once in place, he "inflated" it with 4 ounces of water.

As mentioned earlier, the function of the balloon is twofold. First it inflates the colon to move the posterior (outside) wall of the rectum out of the range of the proton beam. Secondly, it helps to immobilize the prostate by forcing it up against the pelvic bone. This ensures the prostate is always in the same position before daily radiation treatment. This day, they were doing it in order to prepare me for the CT scan.

While lying snugly in the pod, with my balloon firmly in place, the technician began pouring warm polyurethane between the PVC pod and the sheet on which I was lying. This produced a mold that conformed to my body and would essentially keep me motionless while I was being treated. I actually found it to be quite comfortable.

Secure in my newly fabricated immobilization pod, I was wheeled into the CT scan room. During the next 20 minutes they took 98 pictures or "slices" of my anatomy in the prostate region. These pictures would be used to produce a 3-dimensional "hologram" of my prostate, which the oncologists, physicists and dosimetrists would use to plan my treatment.

This information is also used to construct two custom-made focusing devices called an aperture and a bolus, which, along with a selected energy-modulator, would be used to conform the proton beam to the precise target area. This area, I was told, included the prostate, the capsule surrounding the prostate, the nearby seminal vesicles and an extra half inch of margin around the whole "package."

With pod and CT scan completed, I met with my case manager and requested a start date that would allow me to be home for Christmas. Despite the patient overload, Sharon made some adjustments and arranged a start date that would have me home by December 22nd. That is just one of the dozens of ways the people at LLUCC went out of their way to accommodate my needs and make me feel like a special patient. I later learned from others that they all felt the same way.

Note: Being claustrophobic, I was a bit leery about being in an immobilization pod and having a CT scan. Neither of these caused me any discomfort, and the entire process was uneventful.

Where Will We Live for Eight Weeks?

The next challenge I faced was finding a place to stay in the Loma Linda area for my two-month out-patient treatment period. Again, the folks at LLUCC came through. They gave me a packet of information about apartment complexes that offered special rates and two-month furnished rentals to LLUCC patients. They also gave me a stack of hand-outs on things to do while visiting "The Inland Empire," as the San Bernardino/Riverside county area is known. I was so impressed. These people thought of everything.

I didn't fully understand the meaning of the *Make Man Whole* mission at first. But the more time I spent with the staff, the clearer the meaning became. As a Seventh-day Adventist Institution, Loma Linda University Medical Center embraces the Christian philosophy that the human body is the temple of God. Although the senior administrative people at the hospital are members of the Seventh-day Adventist Church, the medical and support staff represent people from all religious backgrounds and beliefs. Yet all seem to embrace the *Make Man Whole* philosophy, which is to restore man to wholeness, physically, emotionally, and spiritually.

At no time during my two-month stay did I feel any pressure to learn more about or participate in any Seventh-day Adventist activities. However, their spiritual presence was felt, and it turned out to be a large factor in my positive experience at LLUCC and in my healing.

I chose to stay at the Redlands Lawn and Tennis Club (RLTC), which was three miles down the road from the hospital. The RLTC had beautiful furnished apartments, and the grounds and location were superb. Since my wife, Pauline, would be joining me, along with other visitors from the East, I felt having a comfortable, roomy apartment was important.

How Will We Spend Our Time?

Now that I was committed to spending two months in Southern California away from friends, children, and support systems, I began to wonder how my wife and I would spend our time. I needed to be at the hospital each day, five days a week for my daily treatments. I felt I couldn't wander far off. Would I be terribly bored after the first few days?

LLUCC pays particular attention to patients' physical and emotional needs as many other proton centers do today. All proton treatment patients are automatically enrolled in the, state-of-the-art, Drayson Center for Recreation and Wellness, located on the campus. This six-acre facility includes four tennis courts, indoor basketball courts and track, two enormous pools, five racquetball courts, and thousands of square feet of fitness equipment.

Numerous psychosocial programs have been established to help meet some of the emotional and social needs of patients. I vowed to participate in some of these. After all, I wanted more of the "magic" I experienced at the support group meeting the night before.

Overflowing with information and enriched with new knowledge, I flew home confident, optimistic, and awaiting my start date – Oct. 25, 2000.

CHAPTER 9

My Treatment Begins

"He who is outside the door has already got a good part of his journey behind him."

– Dutch proverb

A Warm California Reception?

My wife and I flew to California on Tuesday, Oct. 24, 2000, to get settled in our new temporary apartment. We landed in Los Angeles, picked up our rental car, and drove east toward Loma Linda. Traffic was horrific, and the 70-mile trip lasted almost three hours. We arrived at Redlands about 9 p.m., parked the car, and carried our gear up to our second-floor apartment. Somehow, I managed to sprain my back in the process. It was hot – about 85°F – and the air conditioning in our new apartment was broken. Not a great start.

The next morning there was a nasty note on the windshield of my rental car reminding me that I parked in the reserved space of another tenant. How was I to know the spaces were reserved?

We'd been there less than 24 hours; we experienced a horrible traffic jam; I sprained my back; our air conditioning didn't work; and I managed to "tick-off" one of my new neighbors. A bad omen?

Treatment Number 1

My first of 38 treatments was on Wednesday, Oct. 25, 2000, at 1:30 p.m. Pauline was invited to observe. This both surprised and delighted me. Despite all my research, I really didn't know what to expect that first day, and neither did my wife.

My instructions were to consume 16 ounces of water about 20 minutes before the procedure in order to fill my bladder. This helps to stretch the bladder and lift it off the prostate and out of the range of the proton beam. I dutifully complied and drank the water.

Tip: Drink the water. The bladder and prostate are somewhat like a hot air balloon sitting on top of a passenger gondola. When the hot air balloon is full of warm air, it lifts and rises off the gondola.

We were escorted to a changing room where I was told to disrobe and put on a hospital johnny. I could leave my socks on. Somehow that comforted me – but I don't know why. Pauline joined me in the changing room, to provide company and encouragement. A few minutes later, the door to the changing room opened and the previously treated patient, dressed in his johnny, entered – a slightly awkward moment with Pauline there. It was time for my first treatment.

Pauline and I walked down the corridor and entered Gantry 3. We were greeted by three radiation therapists – Tim, Nick, and Barbara, all beaming with welcoming smiles. I remember thinking, "Sure – it's easy for them to smile – I'm the one having 250 million electron volts shot into my private parts."

I was asked to climb into my pod, which had already been installed on the gantry treatment table. "How do you know this is my pod?" I asked. They told me my name was written on it and it was bar coded. The bar code was scanned into the computer in the gantry control room.

Pinching the back of my johnny to hold it closed, lest I show three strangers my best angle, I gingerly climbed into the pod. The smile on the lead therapist's face told me that perhaps everybody is modest at first. Later, I would find myself bounding into the pod with an untied johnny flapping in the breeze and my "better side" fully exposed for all to see.

The pod fit perfectly, almost like it was made for me – but then, it was.

I was asked to roll over on my left side and was presented with my first "official" balloon – not so bad, but a little embarrassing in

122

front of my wife, especially when they filled it with water from two syringes.

As instructed, I rolled onto my back again and they made an initial adjustment to my position in the pod by tugging on the sheet under me. I was conscious of the water-filled balloon in its "resting place." It felt a little unnatural at first, but not uncomfortable.

Next, the pod and platform assembly was slid to the center of the treatment apparatus, and the entire 94-ton gantry began to rotate in order to position the low-energy X-ray equipment above me. At first, I had the sensation that my pod was rotating, and the room was stationary. I found myself hanging on so I wouldn't fall out. I quickly adapted to that phenomenon.

So, there I was 3,000 miles from home, at a hospital in Southern California, lying in a pod, a water balloon in my butt, a sheet covering me, cantilevered into the center of a three-story high, white, cylindrical 94-ton gantry, with two radiation devices pointed at my pelvic region, about to have billions of protons shot into my prostate. I remember thinking, "What the hell am I doing here?"

At this point Pauline broke down and cried. It seemed to hit her all at once: My diagnosis with prostate cancer; all the research, the phone calls, a two-month move to California; my lying helplessly in this "coffin-like" device, surrounded by hospital technicians dressed in white; and this giant "Star Wars" machinery rotating around me. She was suddenly struck with thoughts of the mortality of her partner and best friend of 35 years. Death was something we never discussed, or even thought about, because we considered ourselves young, healthy, and physically fit.

With some comforting by the gentle and caring therapists, Pauline regained her composure, and she and the technicians moved behind a radiation barrier. Suddenly there was a short "zap" from the X-ray machine above me. The technicians then pressed a button and the huge gantry rotated 90 degrees. Back behind the barrier and another quick "zap." These low-energy X-rays were taken from the top and the side to find pre-mapped points on my pelvic bone to ensure that I was in precisely the right spot before the high-energy proton radiation beam was introduced.

While the orthogonal X-rays were being analyzed by the computer, one of the technicians installed three more devices in the gantry machinery that were specifically designed and constructed, or selected for me: the energy modulator, the Cerrobend-lead alloy aperture and the jeweler's wax bolus. These three devices, which help focus the proton beam precisely to the target volume, were bar coded and had to be scanned before the computers would allow the technicians to call for the proton beam.

The size and geometry of these devices were determined from the CT scan and resulting hologram made of my prostate. The purpose was to ensure that the proton beam was delivered to my prostate, the capsule surrounding my prostate, my seminal vesicles and an extra half-inch margin around the entire package. This is done to tolerances of about plus or minus a millimeter. Extraordinary technology!

Based on the information gathered by the two low-energy X-rays, the computer determined the final adjustment that needed to be made to my pod and platform, to place me in the proper position for the proton beam to do its work.

The technicians made this final adjustment and then called in the attending radiation oncologist to check all the settings. The doctor came in, checked the information on the computer screen and the position of the pod in the gantry, and gave his approval to call for the beam. This procedure, including the doctor's final check, would be repeated 37 more times.

Next, I heard Tim Holmes, the lead technician, who looked more like a movie star than a radiation therapist, pick up the intercom and tell the accelerator control room, "Gantry 3 is ready for the beam" (Tim and his girlfriend, Andrea, would later become friends).

Tim told me that everything was ready, and that everyone needed to leave the room. "Does that include me?" I quipped. "No," Tim chuckled, "You'll have to stay here."

Now I was alone in the gantry, and it was totally silent. I remember feeling instantly frightened – and inexplicably sad. Tears began to flow as I lay there helplessly in a custom-made pod, with a balloon in my butt, and surrounded by all this machinery. I knew from the orientation tour that the technicians and my wife were in the Gantry 3 control room and were watching me on a TV monitor. I quickly regained my composure so I wouldn't embarrass myself.

Three or four minutes went by and nothing happened. "What do I do now?" I thought. I began to pray. Then I thought about all the research I had done, all the books and articles I had read, the Internet searches, and the interviews. Yes, the interviews! I had spoken with

56 men who had chosen this treatment. "They all can't be wrong," I thought. The more I concentrated on the work I had done that led me to this place, the more I relaxed. I wiped away the tears, smiled, and thought, "Thank you, God."

Suddenly the energy modulator wheel began to spin. The whirring sound was eerie, but befitting this "Star Wars" movie set I was in. I knew this meant the beam was coming next, and I found myself getting rigid, as if someone were about to punch me in the stomach. But I willed myself to relax. I didn't want to do anything that might move my prostate even a fraction of an inch.

Then I heard the first beep, followed by another, and another – about one a second. This was the Geiger counter-type device that confirms the beam is being properly delivered. I remember counting the beeps to estimate the duration of the treatment. It was just about 60 seconds.

The beeping stopped, and the energy modulator whirring slowed and eventually stopped. I felt nothing – no pain, no discomfort, no burning sensation. It was over. My first treatment was completed. I felt energized; I felt relieved; I was happy; and I knew then I had made the right choice.

Pauline and the Gantry 3 crew came back into the room and congratulated me – as if I had anything to do with what had just happened.

"OK. Mr. Marckini," Tim said. "Party's over – time to give us back the balloon. Please roll over on your left side." I complied and he removed the balloon after draining the water into a small syringe-like reservoir.

I climbed out of the pod, thanked the radiation therapists, and walked back to the dressing room with Pauline. Once there, we hugged, and I said, "We made the right decision."

Each day it was the same routine: Drink the water, climb into the pod, receive my balloon, and get zapped. Nothing to it! I was into the routine, and it was a piece of cake.

Early Treatment Time

I quickly learned that being treated in the middle of the day was undesirable. It didn't allow me to schedule golf, or for us to go sightseeing in the beautiful Inland Empire. So, I asked the manager of the proton treatment unit if it were possible to shift to an earlier time slot. He suggested that I take it up with the radiation therapists in Gantry 3. I did as he suggested, and a few days later, I had a 7:20 a.m. time slot. This was perfect because it gave us the entire day to have fun. It also gave us a three-day weekend (I was finished for the week early Friday morning), and plenty of time to explore a large part of Southern California.

I didn't know how lucky I was to get this early time slot until later, when I learned that, as the day progressed, the probability of the schedule becoming disrupted by late arrivals, occasional equipment problems or computer glitches increased somewhat.

Golf, Guitar, and Grazing

The early time slot allowed me to complete treatment before breakfast and then have the rest of the day to exercise and play.

I learned there are about 30 golf courses within short driving distance of Loma Linda. The Redlands Country Club, one of the oldest golf courses in Southern California, was about five minutes from our apartment. This private club offers LLUCC outpatients temporary memberships at a reasonable price. So, it looked like my golf needs would be taken care of.

Next, I searched for and found a music store and guitar teacher to help me improve my skills with that uncompromising six-stringed instrument.

The Redlands, CA, Chamber of Commerce and the local AAA were most helpful in providing us with information about local tourist attractions, maps, and driving directions.

There are lots of excellent restaurants in the area. Pauline and I set out to visit each one of them. We never had to travel any farther than San Bernardino, Redlands, or Riverside for superb dining that would satisfy the taste of even the most discriminating gourmet.

My Routine

For the next two months I arose at 6:30 a.m., showered, drank my 24 ounces of water (16 ounces were required, but the "recovering engineer" wanted a little insurance), had my treatment, and was back at the apartment in time to make coffee and awaken my wife to plan a fun day of golf, tennis or sightseeing. This is hardly the scenario one would expect for treating a life-threatening disease.

Each patient is encouraged to meet with his radiation oncologist weekly. I met with my doctor on Wednesdays, but since the treatment was going so smoothly, I rarely had anything of consequence to talk about. I was fascinated by proton treatment, so I used the meetings as opportunities to learn as much as I could about proton treatment technology.

Pauline joined me for many of the meetings, and her questions were answered as well. I found myself looking forward to my weekly meetings.

The Nutritionist

During the first week of treatment, patients are asked to meet with the Department of Radiation Medicine nutritionist. While it's not essential to change your diet during treatment, avoiding certain foods could help prevent some temporary, minor intestinal problems, such as diarrhea.

Pauline and I met with Stella, a wonderful Jamaican lady with a smile that won us over before she spoke a word. Soft gospel music was playing on her portable stereo, and I had a good feeling about the meeting we were about to have.

We learned that Stella was a Seventh-day Adventist, and as such, she followed the Adventist diet regimen, which is largely vegetarian, with other restrictions such as no caffeine or alcohol. Thankfully, she didn't tell me I had to temporarily curtail my meat, caffeine or wine during treatment. Eliminating meat, I could possibly handle, but giving up breathing would be easier than skipping my morning coffee.

Stella gave me some information on a healthy diet for life, with some specific suggestions for minor diet changes during treatment, including avoiding such foods as nuts, prunes and green leafy vegetables.

I can't say that I strictly followed Stella's recommendations during treatment, but I did make a few changes.

My diet was generally healthy. I rarely ate red meat, eggs, or butter at the time. Chicken, turkey, and fish were regular staples. Salads, fresh vegetables, and bean soups were also a part of my regular diet. Breakfast typically consisted of a banana, oat, bran or wheat cereals, and of course, coffee. A man needs a few vices in his life!

I later learned that many proton patients have life-changing experiences at Loma Linda that go beyond being cured of cancer. Often this begins with Stella's tips on diet and nutrition, and her explanation of how important this is to our general health and longevity. Most patients, I learned, complete their treatment leaving with a commitment to a healthier overall lifestyle. We were no exception.

Based on subsequent reading and research, I've since made several changes in my diet and will discuss this in later chapters.

Emotional Fitness

Psychological or emotional health has been shown to enhance physical health and strengthen the immune system, which helps prevent disease and hasten the healing process.

As mentioned earlier, *radiation works by damaging the cancer cells' DNA, preventing the cells from reproducing. Healthy cells damaged by radiation typically repair themselves and reproduce, while the damaged cancer cells eventually die off. Clearly both processes – healthy cell repair and cancer cell death – are enhanced by a healthy emotional state and a positive mental attitude.*

Scientific studies have shown that emotional and psychological factors can positively or negatively impact the immune system's ability to fend-off diseases of all kinds, including cancer.

As mentioned earlier, the cancer center had established a social work department within radiation medicine as part of their effort to provide emotional/psychological support to patients while in treatment.

I've often been critical of the over-dependency of our culture on psychologists, psychiatrists and psychotherapists, and the small percentage of these practitioners who actually do their patients any good (I've seen some people harmed by their psychotherapists).

However, I *do* believe there's a place for competent psychologists, psychiatrists and social workers in our society.

The psychosocial programs at Loma Linda are amazingly effective. At the heart of these programs is the Wednesday night support-group meeting.

When I was doing my research and interviewing proton patients, the Wednesday night support-group meetings were frequently mentioned. I heard, "You must attend," or, "Don't miss a single one." I put that advice aside, because of my belief that, "real men don't do support groups." I had visions of 50 people sitting in a circle, holding hands and singing Kumbaya. I couldn't have been more wrong. My experience while there for my consult convinced me of that.

Since my treatments started on a Wednesday, I had the opportunity to attend my second Wednesday night support group meeting – the first for Pauline. We arrived just after 5:30, and at Pauline's suggestion, planned to stay for an hour and then go out to dinner. We helped ourselves to some refreshments and entered the room. Once again, it was packed with about 90 people sitting around rectangular tables, and a few seated on folding chairs randomly placed in any available space. There were no empty chairs, and others were standing, so we decided to stand near the door so we could make our quiet exit.

The mood in the room was festive. People were laughing; and that didn't make sense to Pauline, even though I had explained to her my experience of this meeting two weeks before.

Gerry Troy stood up and introduced himself. With a calm and sincere voice, he welcomed all of us, reminded us to help ourselves to some refreshments, and told us the location of the restrooms. The latter, I learned is important, as urinary urgency is a common temporary side effect of *any* radiation delivered to the pelvic region.

Gerry then made some announcements about group activities. Next, he read a poem and a couple of jokes, all sent to him by former patients, expressly for this meeting. These were well received, and we found ourselves laughing with the rest of the group.

He then asked if there were any alumni in the audience. Seven hands went up. He called on one of them – a gentleman about 60 years old from Arizona named Richard – who stood up and told his story. Richard began by announcing his pretreatment PSA and Gleason score. Then he talked about how his prostate cancer was discovered; his shock and disbelief; the meeting with his urologist who recommended surgery; his investigation of the alternatives; his discovery of proton treatment; the help he received from former proton patients; his physician's unprofessional behavior when he heard Richard had chosen proton treatment ("Find yourself another urologist when you return!"); his wonderful experience of both treatment and his two-month stay in Southern California. He then reported his most recent PSA, 0.9, which drew spontaneous applause from the audience.

This process was repeated six more times. The PSAs, Gleason scores, and home states varied, but the stories were very similar: They all looked beyond their urologist's first recommendation; did their homework; investigated their options; got help from former proton patients; chose proton therapy; and had a wonderful experience.

Gerry then asked if there were any visitors who were not patients. Surprisingly, four hands went up. One at a time people stood up to tell their story. They had been recently diagnosed with prostate cancer and were investigating their options. Two were from California and two from out of state. They were there for consults with radiation oncologists and to see firsthand what proton treatment was all about. They stood, reported their numbers, and talked about where they were in their decision-making process. Each was there with his wife, or significant other, which was the case for most of the other men in the room. Thank God for this support from our partners in life.

Next Gerry asked if there were any newbies present. I raised my hand, along with about 12 other men. One at a time we told our story. We ranged in age from early 50s to late 70s and hailed from several U.S. states – one was from Canada. One of the 12 had been fitted for his pod but hadn't begun treatment. The rest of us were in the early stages of our treatment. I found myself comfortably talking to this group of "brothers," and I drew a few chuckles when I told them about the 56 interviews.

Others who were in treatment raised their hands and offered comments, observations, poems, and songs they had written about their experience of the pod and the rectal balloon. These two subjects seemed to receive a lot of attention, always in a humorous vein.

I noticed one young woman sitting in the room, and one side of her face appeared to be sunburned. I learned that she was being treated at the proton center for an inoperable tumor on the optic nerve of her left eye. Others in the room were there for tumors on the brain or eye. And one was being treated for macular degeneration. Most who raised their hands and spoke that night were prostate cancer patients. I later learned that, at that time, prostate cancer patients represented about 65 percent of the patients treated at the proton center.

A guest speaker made a presentation that evening. It was Dr. Dan Miller, chief physicist at the medical center. He used overhead slides and a white board to explain in great detail how protons are generated; how they are intentionally "spilled" from the accelerator and directed to the treatment rooms; how the narrow beam is expanded; and how the customized devices shape the beam precisely to each patient's targeted area. Dr. Miller had invited questions at the beginning of his presentation, and the crowd was not bashful. He answered dozens of questions during his talk and for about 20 minutes after it ended.

I looked at my watch and discovered it was 8:30 p.m. We had been there for 3 hours and it seemed like 15 minutes! "If all the Wednesday night support group meetings are like this one," I thought, "I'm not going to miss one of them." They were – and I didn't.

My experience of the psychosocial programs at LLUCC, such as the Wednesday night support group, was a major factor in a life-changing decision I would later make, to form a support group that would become international in scope and impact the lives of thousands of people.

Gerry Troy's dream was to take the programs he helped pioneer at Loma Linda and take them to other medical institutions. He left Loma Linda and helped establish a similar, successful patient program at the University of Florida Health Proton Therapy Institute in Jacksonville, Florida. Other proton centers, I have learned, have established similar psychosocial support programs to the substantial benefit of their patients.

Tip: Make sure you participate in the patient support programs when you're in treatment. They're an integral part of your treatment and the healing process. And, they're a lot of fun.

Physical Fitness

Another thing I learned early in my treatment is that staying physically fit greatly benefits the immune system and aids the healing process. A strong immune system also helps prevent cancer recurrence. This bears repeating.

> *Tip: Staying physically fit greatly benefits the patient while in treatment and aids the healing process. It also strengthens the immune system which helps prevent cancer recurrence.*

When I sat through the orientation session during my first visit, I was given a large packet of information on a wide range of subjects including places to stay in the community during treatment, points of interest, technical papers on proton therapy, maps of the area and other general information. I was reminded that, in California, at 57 years of age, I had already been a "senior citizen" for two years. Not a pleasant thought for me, as I considered myself *"approaching* middle age."* Nevertheless, there were benefits to being a senior at Loma Linda. Among them were discounts at the hospital cafeteria and preferred parking spaces at the medical center.

Another part of the packet of information I received was a certificate that authorized my wife and me to use the expansive, state-of-the-art recreation and wellness facility on the university campus, called the Drayson Center. This complex is named in honor of Dr. Ronald and Grace Drayson, who provided the lead gift that was used to help build the center.

The $16 million complex serves students, faculty, and patients. The Drayson Center's mission is to provide opportunities for enhancement of the quality of life within this community through a wide variety of social, recreational, and health-building activities, all consistent with LLUMC's mission, *To Make Man Whole*.

Pauline and I were already in reasonably good physical condition. We both exercised regularly and had been following a generally healthy lifestyle.

We were encouraged to visit the Drayson Center and take advantage of all it had to offer while I was there for treatment – and we did. Each day we would visit the center and spend about 90 minutes working out. We began our workout by spending a half hour on one of the treadmills. Then we switched to the fitness equipment to do upper and lower body exercises. We found ourselves looking forward to our daily routine at the Drayson Center, and during our eight-week stay we increased both our physical strength and our endurance.

Following our late morning workout, we fell into another routine: Eating lunch at the hospital cafeteria. Seventh-day Adventists take a healthy diet very seriously, and that naturally extends to the hospital cafeteria.

'Stealth' Health

Without realizing it, I had been gently led down three very important paths. Within the first few days of my stay, I was eating a more healthful diet; I was exercising daily; and I was participating in programs aimed at nurturing my emotional well-being.

When I returned home in December 2000, I was stronger, healthier, and more physically fit. And, as it turned out, I had a new perspective on spirituality and my faith.

Little wonder that proton patients go through "withdrawal" as they near the end of their treatment.

'Lover's Groan' and other Short-Term Side Effects

During the first few weeks of treatment, my wife and I continued our normal intimacies as we were told we could. Around week six however, I noticed a burning sensation deep in my groin, during sex. This became somewhat more noticeable as my treatments progressed.

My doctor explained that my prostate was being irradiated every day by the powerful proton beam; that the discomfort I was experiencing was normal; and that it would dissipate after treatment ended.

When I compared notes with other men in treatment, I learned that many had similar experiences. One jokingly referred to this unique experience as "lover's groan," and the term seemed to stick.

As predicted, the discomfort disappeared a few weeks after treatment ended.

About the same time the "lover's groan" appeared, I began to experience some slight urinary burning and increased urgency to urinate. At night I found myself having to make three or four bathroom trips. During the day it was worse. At times I couldn't go much more than a half hour before having to visit the restroom.

That wasn't so bad, but things got a little more complicated when I was playing golf one day about seven weeks into treatment.

Really Strange Golfer

I went to Oak Valley Golf Club in Beaumont by myself that day and was matched up with three women. There were only two restrooms on the course, and I knew I was going to get into trouble as the urinary urgency was just about at its peak, with relief stops needed about every 20 minutes. Fortunately, the golf course was mature and heavily wooded.

At first, I managed my relief by lagging behind after finishing a hole, pretending I left a club or golf glove on the previous green. Then I would sneak into the bushes as the other three walked ahead. As the match progressed and we became friends, the three of them began to wait for me out of courtesy, denying me my much-needed comfort break.

I was a high handicap golfer, so I often hit my fair share of balls to landing areas other than the fairway. But never had I intentionally directed balls into the woods – until that day. At least once on every hole I would wind up and crack one deep into the brush or over a hill behind a sand trap, and then gingerly trot after it to get my blessed relief.

My golf partners must have thought it a bit odd when I frequently lined up about 45 degrees from the direction of the green and swatted one deep into the woods. I suspect they talk about that "crazy guy" to this day.

Things were a little easier off the golf course, but I *did* realize that my fellow prostate cancer radiation patients and I had one thing in common: We knew exactly where every public restroom was located in San Bernardino County. At one Wednesday night meeting,

134

one of the patients produced a map of the community with every public restroom identified within a 5-square-mile radius of the hospital. The audience laughed uncontrollably – and then they all requested copies.

The urinary urgency and slight burning issues were short lived. My doctor prescribed Pyridium Plus, a drug used to treat urinary tract irritation. This took care of the problem until it disappeared on its own a few weeks after treatment ended. This medication has an interesting side effect – it turns your urine to a bright day-glow red color. Not a problem unless you are at a urinal and someone catches sight of your fluorescent discharge. This earned me a few strange looks in public restrooms.

CHAPTER 10

The Fun Part of Spending Eight Weeks in Southern California

"A truly happy person is one who can enjoy the scenery on a detour."

– Unknown

Getting into the Swing of Things

Loma Linda provides a list of dozens of furnished rooms and apartments to stay in during treatment. As mentioned earlier, Pauline and I chose the Redlands Lawn and Tennis Club, a condo/apartment facility, three miles down the road from the hospital with tennis courts, swimming pool, and exercise room in a beautifully landscaped, gated community.

We enjoyed the "freedom" of apartment living for eight weeks and made friends with two of our neighbors. One couple was a young man who was a civilian employee of the Department of Defense and his wife Rene, a German national who was learning to speak English. They were lots of fun. Her "bloopers" with the English language provided much entertainment while we were together.

It took me quite a while, for example, to understand the word "reeseep," which she used several times in a conversation one day. Finally, I had to ask her, "Rene, what is this word, 'reeseep?'" She said indignantly, "Reeseep, spelled r-e-c-i-p-e, reeseep!" There were many more of these gems in her vocabulary.

Rene also picked up some slang and some colloquialisms along the way. One was the term "gang bang." She thought it meant, "a funny event." After a water pipe broke in her apartment one day, the landlord sent a plumber, a carpenter, and a clean-up crew to fix things. At dinner that night she told us, "You should have seen it – the plumber, the carpenter, and the clean-up guys – we had a real gang bang in my apartment today."

Pauline spent much of her time reading, walking, and learning to knit. The latter provided me with much amusement, as she chose a complex pattern for her first project and managed to disassemble it and start over about 30 times during our stay, effectively "wearing out" the yarn.

The Drayson Center occupied most of our mornings. Golf, guitar lessons, sightseeing, reading, tennis, and other activities filled the afternoons. Evenings were often spent exploring the many wonderful restaurants in the Inland Empire.

Golf

A golf practice range was located roughly midway between our apartment and the hospital a mile down the road. The first week of our stay, I loaded my clubs into the rental car; drove there and introduced myself to the teaching pro, Jim Becker, who managed the facility. I told him I was going to be in town for a couple of months and was interested in some lessons. His response was, "Let me guess, you have prostate cancer and you're being treated with protons over at Loma Linda." I was dumbfounded and asked how he knew. He told me he's had a couple hundred golf students come through over the past few years, mostly men in their 50s to their 80s, all with the same story. Jim and I became friends during our stay, and the five lessons I paid for somehow stretched to 12 – at no extra cost. He also provided me with introductions to the pros at several local golf clubs, including two new PGA courses. I played all of them at substantially discounted greens fees, thanks to Jim's introductions. You meet some wonderful people on this journey.

Travel, Tours, Restaurants and More

Pauline and I visited San Diego on one of our three-day weekends. Pauline fell in love with the giant pandas at the San Diego Zoo. I was fascinated by the killer whales on our visit to Sea World.

Our friends, Bob and Barbara Destino live in Mission Viejo, which is about an hour southwest of Loma Linda – with no traffic (All commuting times in Southern California should be multiplied by two or three for rush-hour traffic).

Pauline grew up in Northern Vermont with Barbara, and they have always been close friends. Her husband, Bob, and I have also become friends over the years. We spent an enjoyable three-day weekend playing golf, attending church with them, reminiscing, and catching up on the events of our lives. It was a truly enjoyable weekend. I had to keep reminding myself that I was in California having treatment for a life-threatening disease.

One Sunday morning after church, we decided to visit one of the local attractions listed in the sightseeing pamphlets provided by the LLUCC Social Work Group. The Morey Mansion was only a few blocks from our apartment in Redlands. When we pulled up, we saw only one car in the parking area, suggesting that perhaps it was closed on Sunday. We drove into the parking lot anyway.

No one answered the front doorbell, so we walked around back and were greeted by a lady working in a beautiful garden. I presumed she was one of the groundskeepers and asked if the mansion was open for tours on Sunday. She smiled and told us the mansion hadn't been open for tours for three years. She and her husband purchased the mansion to be their home, and they had spent the past three years restoring it.

I was embarrassed; I apologized for the intrusion and explained how the whole thing happened. To our surprise, she asked if we'd like to see her home now that it had been fully restored. We answered, "Of course!" And then the most amazing thing happened: She suggested we go into the mansion through the back door; go up to the top floor and work our way down, and as soon as she was finished in the yard, she would join us.

At first, we felt uncomfortable walking through the private home of a perfect stranger, but that changed as we began our self-directed tour. The home was extraordinary – fully restored in every detail. The lady joined us, and spent an hour sharing the history of the mansion and the restoration details. To this day, we look back on that event and try to picture something similar happening anyplace else on earth. And we both came to the same conclusion – it could never happen.

The restaurants were superb in the Redlands, San Bernardino, and Riverside areas. We never had time during those eight weeks to visit all of them, but on each return visit, we manage to add more to our list.

In early December we went for a ride on the brand-new rotating tramway gondola, which took us to the top of Mount San Jacinto near Palm Springs. San Jacinto is the second-tallest mountain in Southern California with an elevation of 10,804 feet at the peak. This is not a ride for anyone with acrophobia – like yours truly, but the spectacular view of the Palm Springs area is worth it.

One of the highlights of our stay was a visit to the Crystal Cathedral in Garden Grove. It was a Sunday morning service with Dr. Robert Schuller (since deceased). For years we had watched Dr. Schuller on TV. It was a special treat to be there in the front row – where first-time visitors sat – hearing him preach and listening to the Crystal Cathedral organ and choir.

Tenth Anniversary Celebration

We were fortunate to have been at Loma Linda in November of 2000. This was the 10th anniversary of the opening of the proton treatment center. The celebration was held on Nov. 12, and it lasted all day. There were tours of the facility, chamber music, a luncheon, and a reception hosted by Dr. Lyn Behrens, president and CEO of Loma Linda University Health, the parent organization for the medical center and university. Also hosting the event were Dr. James Slater, the pioneer of proton therapy, and Dr. Jerry Slater, Chairman of the Department of Radiation Medicine.

Later in the day there were presentations given by the above people, welcoming the large gathering of current and former patients as well as faculty, hospital staff, and other guests. Speakers reviewed the history of the project, the challenges, the successes over the past 10 years, and plans for the future. I learned that the tiny proton particle is one of the most powerful forces of nature for curing diseases of all types, and that research is under way at Loma Linda to unleash that power. The only obstacle, I learned, was adequate funding to support that research.

Congressman Jerry Lewis, a key sponsor of the original facility, was unable to attend, but spoke to us by video from his Washington office.

The chief physicist on the project from the FermiLab, Phil Livdahl, also spoke. A humble man, he described the technical challenges and his partnership with Dr. James Slater. He told us that ironically, shortly after the project was completed, he was diagnosed with prostate cancer and became the first prostate cancer patient treated with protons at the new facility. Ten years later he was still cancer free. Years later, I would become friends with this great man, and he would one day join the group that I founded.

One young woman, Jennifer Gardner, told the story of how she was diagnosed at age 17 with an inoperable brain tumor. She and her family were told there was no hope and that she would die. Her aunt, a nurse at Loma Linda, persuaded her to talk with the doctors there about proton treatment. She did, and four years later as she told her story she was cancer free and studying to become a radiation oncologist; there wasn't a dry eye in that packed auditorium.

An organic chemistry professor, Dr. Roy Butler, spoke of his experience with proton treatment for his prostate cancer; how he managed to teach his class at Norwich University 3,000 miles away while being treated; and how he arranged a sabbatical to teach at the University of Redlands and remain in the Loma Linda area for an additional year. Dr. Butler recounted the humorous side of his treatment and quickly had the audience laughing.

During his sabbatical while teaching at the University of Redlands, Roy spent considerable time at LLUCC absorbing everything he could about the technology of proton therapy. Using this information, he produced a comprehensive document explaining the technology in layman's terms. He titled his work, *The Patient Proton*. This important document would later appear on our website, www.protonbob.com.

At the end of the program, the master of ceremonies asked all those in the audience who had benefited from proton therapy to come up to the stage. About 200 of us gathered there. A singer walked up to the microphone and in a booming, baritone voice sang "You'll Never

Walk Alone." As I stood there on stage with the others, the tears began to flow. I wasn't alone. All 200 of us, mostly men who were current and former prostate cancer patients, were standing there with tears of hope in our eyes. And our family members, along with the faculty and staff in the audience had their tissues out too. It was a powerfully emotional experience.

At the conclusion of the program, Dr. J. Lynn Martell walked to the podium and offered a prayer of thanksgiving. During that prayer I remember thinking, Pauline and I should plan to be here for the 20th and 30th anniversaries. How's that for optimism?

Thanksgiving Break and Friends Visit

Halfway through treatment Pauline and I flew home for the long Thanksgiving weekend. Our friends were a little surprised to see me so rested and tanned. I think they expected me to be pale, skinny and bald. On Saturday evening they held a surprise party, where they presented me with a bouquet – of balloons. This "arrangement" consisted of 20 deflated balloons, representing the number of treatments completed, and 18 inflated balloons for the number of treatments remaining. I remember thinking, "What great friends we have!"

My wife stayed home the next two weeks at my request, to make room for several of my friends to visit me in California.

My buddy Steve, from Philadelphia, came first. He's a former high school basketball coach and physical fitness "nut." He thought he'd "died and gone to heaven" when I took him to the Drayson Center.

Steve and I are on opposite sides of the political spectrum and at that time the presidential election of 2000 was still in contention. The ballots were being recounted in Florida for the second or third time. We had many heated discussions during his visit, and we're still good friends to this day.

Following Steve's visit, four friends from the East Coast arrived: Joe, Paul, Ed and Frank. They brought their golf clubs, and we have photographs and memories of their visit that will last a lifetime.

142

While they were at Loma Linda, I arranged for them to tour the proton treatment center and to observe one of my 7:20 a.m. treatments. After the tour, all five of us crowded into the changing room where I slipped into my hospital johnny. Then they accompanied me into the gantry where I climbed into my pod to prepare for my daily dose of protons. All the while, my friend Ed was snapping photos with his digital camera. Here I prepared a little surprise for them.

My friend Joe Bruno and I have played practical jokes on each other over the years. It was Joe who arranged for the unique balloon bouquet at home. Prior to my friends' visit, I had rehearsed some dialogue with Tim, the lead radiation therapist who would be inserting my rectal balloon that morning.

All four of my friends were huddled together on one side of the gantry while the three therapists were going about their business. Tim asked me to roll over on my left side, in order to allow him to insert the ignominious balloon. Just as he began the process, I leaned over my right shoulder and asked, "Tim, all the time you've been shoving the balloon up there, I never asked. What do you call this procedure?" He replied, "Mr. Marckini, we call this the *Bruno Procedure*." That caught my friends completely off guard, and certainly lightened things up. I was later told the laughter could be heard in the Level B waiting room a good distance away.

Weekly Note to Friends

Another way I occupied my time during those eight weeks was by writing weekly status reports to friends on my computer and distributing them by email. I shared, not only the status of my treatment regimen and the things Pauline and I were doing to occupy our time, but also some of my observations of living in Southern California for eight weeks.

I tried to find the humor in what was happening to me and around me and share it in my reports. My friends were entertained by these notes and they shared them with others. Each week I was asked to add more email addresses to my distribution list. By the time I completed treatment, I was sending copies of my weekly notes to 75 people. Here is an excerpt from one report where I was making some observations of life in Southern California:

Driving down the highway the other day, I noticed a sign. It said, "Fine for illegally driving in the carpool lane: $271." Now try to stretch your imagination. Why . . . how . . . under what conditions could any rational human being or governmental agency choose a fine of $271 for driving in a carpool lane? Why not $300, or $250, or even $275? But $271?? Only in California!

Did you know that there were 261 earthquakes in California last week? This is a fact. Check out this website: http://quake.wr.usgs.gov/recenteqs/. Most of these are only detectable by seismic equipment, but the fact remains – this place is movin' and shakin'. I knew California had more quakes than most other states, but I had no idea there were that many. Why would anybody want to live here?

We saw a nice holiday scene around the corner from our apartment this week . . . a Christmas tree on a front lawn decorated entirely with Budweiser beer cans. Only in California.

One of the popular radio shows out here is the Phil Hendrie Show. He invites controversial characters to call in, and then for other callers to challenge them. Last Tuesday a car dealer from Beverly Hills called to complain about the Stage 2 power alert in California. He was upset that he had to turn off the power to his Christmas manger scene at his dealership. Seems he had the infant in the manger outfitted with a mechanical arm that handed out free drink certificates for a local bar. They really know how to celebrate the spirit of Christmas out here.

Another guy called in and told Phil that he was suing his wife because she made him buy leather pants to wear to an outdoor rock concert. They were sitting on metal folding chairs; the pants ripped in the seat; and he apparently froze his private parts. He claims this has interfered with his ability to have a connubial relationship with his wife and is suing her for lack of consortium. Only in California.

And how about the weird names Southern Californians give to their cities – Temecula, La Jolla, Topanga, Alhambra, Chula Vista, Coalinga, and Rancho Cucamonga. What ever happened to real "nuts-and-bolts" American city names like Flint, Bayonne, and Malden? I'm telling you, they're nuts out here.

144

Christmas in Loma Linda

Near the end of my treatment, we were approaching the Christmas holidays. I'll never forget what happened at a Wednesday night support-group meeting in mid-December. Dr. Lynn Martell, who attended most of the meetings, stood up and asked the group of a hundred or so, "How many of you will still be here during the Christmas holidays?" A bunch of hands went up. Next, he said, "No one should spend Christmas away from home in a lonely apartment. I'd like to invite you all to come to my home and have Christmas dinner with me and my family."

I was flabbergasted. It felt like a scene from "It's a Wonderful Life." I tried to imagine a senior administrative official at a hospital back in Boston inviting dozens of patients to his home for Christmas dinner.

About 65 people accepted Lynn's invitation and spent Christmas with the Martell family. I didn't learn until later that Lynn's invitation that night was spontaneous. He hadn't discussed it with his wife. I could not imagine telling my wife, "Oh honey, I just invited 65 strangers to spend Christmas day with us. What will you be serving for dinner?"

Dr. Martell and his lovely wife, Karen, continued this tradition for 16 years. They've had as many as 90 patients and their families in their home for Christmas dinner. They set up tables in every room of their house, including bedrooms, and a bathroom! Every year the guests reported they had a terrific meal and a great time.

Let's Form a Support Group

During treatment, I became friends with several men who were also receiving treatment for prostate cancer. This included a recently retired Northwest Airlines pilot from Washington state; a brilliant chemistry professor from Vermont; a magazine publisher from Chicago; a scientist and professional photographer from Washington state; and a deputy district attorney for San Bernardino County; a county commissioner for Umatilla County, Oregon, and others.

As we approached the end of our eight-week treatment period, we talked about ways to keep in touch, to maintain our friendships, and to communicate about side effects, post-treatment PSAs and other factors involving our treatment and healing. I recommended we form an email support group. No one else would have to know. After all, "real men" don't join support groups. This would be our own little secret club, like in the Robin Williams movie, "Dead Poet's Society."

Little did we know at the time, that this little venture was about to take on a life of its own.

CHAPTER 11

Life After Proton Treatment

"Life changes very quickly, in a very positive way, if you let it."

– Lindsey Vonn

As I update this chapter it's more than 19 years since I received proton therapy. If one were to ask me if my life has changed as a result of my treatment for prostate cancer, I would say, "Are you kidding? The answer is *yes – profoundly –* and all for the better!"

Side Effects

As far as side effects are concerned, I can truly say they were minimal and temporary. The short-term urinary urgency and slight burning during urination left me within a few weeks after treatment ended. Bladder control is normal. There has been one positive benefit of my treatment – my prostate has shrunk in size from the proton radiation. I no longer get up at night to visit the bathroom. And thankfully, our sex life is as good as it was before treatment.

When the prostate is removed during surgery, there is no more ejaculate during climax for those who are fortunate enough to remain potent. Similarly, when the prostate is bombarded with radiation, it's common for the volume of ejaculate to be significantly reduced, often to zero. Most of us don't see this as a problem as it doesn't interfere with the enjoyment of the sexual experience. And some see it as a distinct advantage!

147

The radiation "tan mark" entry point on each of my hips roughly conformed to the profile of the lead alloy aperture used to shape the beam during treatment. I never experienced any sunburn pain or discomfort from these marks, and they disappeared after a few months.

About a year after treatment ended, I experienced some rectal bleeding. I noticed it following a bowel movement. There was about a thimble-full of blood in the bowl. I had been told during treatment that this could happen and that it was normal.

I spoke with my doctor at LLUCC and he explained that the anterior (inside) wall of the rectum can be in the "line of fire" of the proton beam, if it's within the 12 millimeter (half inch) margin around the prostate that's targeted during treatment. The balloon, which inflates the rectum, protects the rest of the circumference of the rectum from seeing any radiation damage.

As this healthy tissue repairs itself, there is a phenomenon called radiation-induced neovascularization. New blood vessels form in the rectal wall, and periodically some blood vessels near the surface leak blood, or a scab will "slough off." This condition is not uncommon, it's self-limiting, and it almost always goes away after a few months. I noticed some blood in my stool about once a month for 18 months, as the condition gradually diminished and disappeared. Once every few years, I might see a spot of blood in my stools. It's a non-event.

Occasionally, I'm told, the bleeding can become a nuisance and may require a painless out-patient procedure called argon plasma coagulation, sometimes referred to as "APC." Rarely does this condition require more than that. Also, with the newly available SpaceOAR hydrogel option for protecting the rectum from radiation, it's possible that the rectal bleeding issue is essentially a thing of the past.

Post-Treatment PSA Trend

Four months after treatment ended, I scheduled a blood test and DRE (digital rectal exam) as directed. The DRE was normal. In fact, my urologist, who was a proton skeptic before I was treated, told me my prostate felt as soft and supple as a much younger man's. "I assume that's good?" I asked. "Of course," was his answer. He told me my prostate had actually shrunk and that it felt normal and healthy. Good news!

Waiting for that first PSA was torture. I remember calling my urologist to learn the results. Many things were going through my mind: *What if it didn't work? What if my PSA is still rising beyond the 8.0 pretreatment level? I never felt any pain or discomfort during treatment – maybe the beam wasn't working, and I didn't know it. Maybe this proton thing is a big scam – after all, no pain no gain, right? And I didn't feel any pain.*

My urologist came on the line and said, "Congratulations. Your PSA is 3.6, right about where it should be."

What a sense of relief! I hadn't had a PSA of 3.6 in years. Even my earliest PSA readings were in the high threes. This was cause for celebration. I called my family and friends, shared the good news and took my wife out to dinner.

Six months later I was disappointed. I was expecting another 50 percent drop, but the reading was 3.3. It was "technically" a drop, but why so little? Was this an indication that I was at the nadir (i.e. the lowest it would go after treatment)? If so, that could spell trouble, as I had read somewhere that the lower the nadir, the better are your chances for long-term cure.

I called my radiation oncologist at Loma Linda. He explained that I had nothing to be concerned about. Post radiation treatment PSA drop is never a straight line. It can be a "roller coaster ride," he explained. He told me that it can plateau, and even temporarily bump up, especially during the first two years following treatment, and, "Not to worry. If it will make you feel any better, retest your PSA in three months instead of waiting six." I did, and my next reading – 13 months after treatment ended – was 2.3. Yes! Cause for another celebration.

I decided to test again in three more months. Again, good news: it had dropped to 1.0. By October 2002, 22 months after treatment, my PSA had fallen to 0.8. "God is good," I thought. All's right with the world!

Keep Your Prostate Quiet

In July 2002, I was scheduled for an annual physical including a PSA test. The previous reading was 1.0. My primary care physician had a substitute nurse that day. His regular nurse was on vacation, so things were a little out of sequence in his office. After the nurse measured my vital signs and ran the EKG, my doctor came in to finish the exam. As he slipped on his rubber glove, I asked him what he was going to do. "Your digital rectal exam," he said. "But you haven't drawn blood yet," I commented. "So what?" he replied.

I told him I had spent a long time researching prostate cancer and PSA on the Internet and I learned anything that stimulates the prostate, such as having sex, a DRE, even riding a bicycle, could cause my PSA to spike resulting in a false reading.

"I've heard that," he said, "but I don't believe it."

I said, "OK, I'll bet you a dollar my PSA will spike at least 30 to 50 percent." He said, "You're on." And he gave me a DRE.

Sure enough, my PSA came in at 1.6 – a 60 percent increase, and I wasn't alarmed. I repeated the PSA test – this time without the DRE – and the number was 0.8. I had convinced my primary care physician that the DRE must be done *after* blood was drawn for PSA, and I had won a dollar. Life was getting better.

Later my PSA would reach a nadir below 1.0 where it has remained.

Tip: Never have your blood drawn soon after having a DRE. Your PSA result will most certainly be elevated, and it will not be representative of your true PSA.

No More Urologist

I think it's interesting to note that the last time I saw my urologist was 19 years ago when I had my first post-treatment PSA. All future PSA testing has been done through my primary care physician, who is one of the finest doctors in the world, as far as I'm concerned.

150

What's interesting is that I've had no need for a urologist for the past 19 years. This is significant. How many radical prostatectomy patients or IMRT patients can say that? Very few, I imagine. And it's not uncommon with proton patients.

Fact is, very few of us former proton patients experience any issues that require the attention of a urologist.

Insurance companies fail to take this into consideration when they complain about the high cost of proton therapy. The follow-up cost of proton therapy has to be significantly lower than with any other form of prostate cancer treatment.

Other Changes in My Life

My life has changed in other ways. I maintained my increased exercise regimen and exercise six days a week. I feel healthier and stronger than I have in years. Although my diet isn't perfect, I find myself eating a generally healthier and more balanced diet, which started with the coaching from Stella, the nutritionist, and was heavily influenced by my subsequent research and readings on diet and health, which I will discuss in later chapters.

Many of the couples we met through proton treatment have become close friends. We exchange emails, phone calls, and even travel and stay at each other's homes.

Invitation to Join Advisory Council

In addition to maintaining contact with patients I met during treatment, I stayed in touch with Dr. J. Lynn Martell, who at that time was vice president of advancement for Loma Linda University Health. I didn't know much about his responsibilities at the time, other than the fact that he was involved in fund raising to support proton therapy research and other programs at the medical center and university.

Shortly after I returned home, I wrote a letter to Dr. Lyn Behrens, CEO of all Loma Linda operations, acknowledging her and the staff for creating an unparalleled healing experience.

In return I received a letter from Dr. Behrens humbly thanking me for taking the time to document my experience and for acknowledging the hard-working people at Loma Linda.

A month later, Dr. Martell sent me a letter inviting me to become a member of the International Advisory Council. I accepted and for 12 years served alongside some very special people, including golfing great, Ken Venturi, the Undersecretary General of the United Nations Ambassador Joseph Verner Reed, the former CEO of Outward Bound, John Raynolds and several other distinguished men. We were all prostate cancer survivors who were treated with proton therapy, and we gladly gave back for the gift we received.

Invitation to Speak at Public Hearing in Hampton, Virginia

In mid-2005, I received a call from Dr. William Harvey, president of Hampton University in Hampton, VA. Hampton University is a progressive 6,200-student institution, founded in 1868, and led by this dynamic visionary. HU is located in a picture-postcard setting on 250 acres with beautiful buildings and breathtaking grounds surrounded by water on three sides. It boasts the first medical physics program in the state and the only one nationally at an historically black college.

They were holding a public hearing to gain community support for a proton treatment center. Dr. Harvey had done his homework. He had researched the technology well, brought in a top-notch physicist, aligned himself with a local oncology group, persuaded the community to donate the land, and gained the support of the mayors of all the surrounding communities. The proposed proton facility would be 96,000 square feet in size and was projected to cost about $133 million.

I was proud to share the podium with other speakers like Dr. Jerry Slater, Chairman of the Department of Radiation Medicine at LLUCC, Dr. Alan Thornton, who at the time was Medical Director at the Midwest Proton Therapy Institute, the Mayor of Hampton, and Don Gothard a former proton patient from Washington, MI.

Dr. Harvey said the facility would be important, medically, for the Commonwealth of Virginia, and would be an economic driver for the community. He envisioned an entire medical institution growing out of the proton treatment facility.

Following is the text of my talk:

My name is Bob Marckini. I am a prostate cancer survivor and a proton therapy patient. I'm pleased to be speaking today in support of the Hampton University Proton Therapy Institute.

Coincidentally, it was five years ago today, August 10th, 2000, when I received a phone call from my urologist. He said, "The biopsy results are in; you have prostate cancer." I didn't hear much of what he said after that, but when my wife and I visited his office a few days later, he told me I was a perfect candidate for surgery, and he'd be happy to do it. All I would have to do is to bank four pints of blood over the next month and I'd be ready to go. The brachytherapist I met with next said I was the perfect candidate for radioactive seeds; and the radiation oncologist told me I was the "poster boy" for External Beam Radiation Therapy. The good news was that I had alternatives. The bad news was that each of them had the potential for complications like blood loss and infection, or side effects like impotence and incontinence.

One thing was for certain: I was <u>not</u> going to choose surgery. Why? Because my older brother went through surgery, two years prior, and I saw what he went through – blood loss (six pints), tubes, drains, catheters, a long recovery, and all that was followed by a complication that required additional surgery. Also, a close friend had chosen surgery and he suffered some pretty nasty side effects. So, I began my research.

I admit that I'm a "recovering engineer." I buried myself in the technical details. And I did all the conventional things: read books, searched the Internet, and met with specialists in each field.

But the heart of my research consisted of interviews with former patients from each treatment modality. I was most interested in side effects and quality-of-life issues. Incontinence concerned me the most. I was 57 years old, and the thought of wearing diapers for the rest of my life frightened me to death.

I learned about proton therapy the way most proton patients do – from a former patient. What I heard was hard to believe: "Non-invasive, no pain, no blood loss, minimal side effects – if any – and cure rates as good as the 'gold standard,' surgery." It sounded too good to be true – and I thought, "Why would anyone undergo major surgery with all the associated risks and side effects, if this painless and effective treatment were available?"

I continued my research, and spoke with former patients who had undergone surgery, brachytherapy (seeds), conventional radiation, and proton therapy. Of all those with whom I spoke, the proton patients were the most enthusiastic – bordering on ecstatic – about their treatment. I interviewed 56 of them. And they confirmed what I heard from the first one – no pain, non-invasive, and minimal to no side effects. The bonus was hearing how they played golf or tennis every day and had a great vacation during their two months of treatment.

I flew to Loma Linda for an orientation tour and consult. And when I saw the technology firsthand and met the wonderful folks at the treatment center, that sealed the deal. I began treatment in mid-October and finished in December 2000.

My treatment was at 7:20 a.m., five days a week. Each treatment lasted just a few minutes. I was out at 7:40 and spent the rest of the day with my wife exercising, playing golf, tennis, or sightseeing. We had a great two-month vacation.

Doctors measure PSA, a protein in the blood, as a relative indicator of the effectiveness of prostate cancer treatment. My pretreatment PSA was 8.0, twice the upper limit of the normal range. Following treatment, as predicted, my PSA began to fall. Today, five years later, my PSA is below 1.0 and I have had no permanent side effects. The quality of my life hasn't changed at all. I couldn't have asked for better results.

While in treatment five years ago, I made new friends – and, there's something stronger and deeper about friendships you make when you share a common bond, like prostate cancer. I was also struck by the type of men who were traveling there from all over the world for proton treatment. They were physicians, scientists, engineers, lawyers, physicists, college professors, and successful businessmen – all intelligent, analytical types who made decisions based on data. This made me feel good about my proton decision.

My new friends and I decided to form a club, so that we could keep in touch and compare notes as we continued our healing journey. We also wanted to maintain our connection with Loma Linda. The psychosocial programs there, combined with their extraordinarily caring attitude, created a wonderful, healing environment – and we didn't want to let that go. I volunteered to lead the group, which I named, "The Brotherhood of the Balloon." The word of our group's formation leaked out, others asked to join – and we grew larger.

Today, we have 2,100 members in 50 states and 17 countries. We have a website with our member database, a discussion board and many other features, including more than a hundred testimonials written by former patients. We have special projects to help members in various ways and we publish a monthly newsletter. We promote proton therapy, both through our website, and by providing members with PowerPoint presentations to take on the road. On any given day, we have members around the world speaking at Lions Clubs, Rotary Clubs, church and community meetings, and at men's prostate cancer support groups. Our reference list consists of dozens of former patients who welcome calls and emails from those who are evaluating treatment options and want to hear firsthand about proton treatment.

In addition to providing support to our members, and promoting proton therapy, we've recently come to realize that we, who benefited from this extraordinary technology, have an obligation to give something back to the institution that saved our lives and maintained the quality of our lives. To that end, we work to both refer patients to Loma Linda and to raise money for proton therapy research. To date, our group has referred more than 1,200 patients, and has raised more than $2.5 million for proton therapy research.

And, we see this as just the beginning. As more proton treatment centers are built, and more and more people discover the healing power of the proton beam, we see our group having much more impact on raising people's awareness of this technology and bringing in significant funding for proton therapy research.

I thought when I received that phone call on August 10th, 2000 – five years ago today – that it was the lowest point in my life. Little did I know that later I would consider that diagnosis to be one of the best things that ever happened to me.

My whole perspective on life and what's important in life has changed; I've had the opportunity to make new and wonderful friends; I've had the opportunity to discover Loma Linda, an extraordinary medical institution, with some of the most competent and dedicated people in the world; and it's given me the privilege of leading a support group and being a part of 2,100 people's lives, the overwhelming majority of whom have had their cancers cured, and the quality of their lives preserved.

Picture this: You're diagnosed with cancer. Your doctor encourages you to have major surgery and announces the possibility of blood loss, infection, and the high probability of impotence and incontinence. Next, imagine you discover a treatment that involves no invasion of your body, no blood loss, no infection, and significantly fewer side effects, if any. You would feel the weight of the world lifted from your shoulders. That's what happens with proton patients. That's what happened to me. And that's the experience of the other 2,100 members of our organization and the tens of thousands of patients who have been treated with proton therapy.

While at Loma Linda I met numerous people, who benefited from proton treatment including Jennifer, a young woman who had a malignant tumor behind her eye. Her doctors said she was untreatable because of the tumor's location. It's now 10 years since her proton therapy, and she's doing fine. I also met Daniel, a young man who had a tumor wrapped around his brain stem, diagnosed when he was 12 years old. After some surgery, doctors told his parents they couldn't get it all, and there was nothing more they could do. That was eight years ago. Proton therapy worked for him too. Today he's a junior in college and he's doing fine.

Proton beam therapy is an extraordinary technology – one that must be shared with the world. I can never thank Drs. Jim and Jerry Slater enough for what they and their team did for me. And as long as I'm alive, I'll do whatever I can to promote proton therapy.

Virginia should count itself fortunate that Hampton University is proposing to establish a proton therapy center. Proton therapy has made a tremendous, positive impact on my life and the lives of the other members of my group. For the sake of the many patients who could benefit from proton therapy, I very much hope that you will approve the Hampton University Proton Therapy Institute. Thank you.

I'm happy to report that Dr. Harvey and Hampton University received approval and support for the project. The Hampton University Proton Treatment Center was designed and constructed over a three-year period and they treated their first patient in October 2010. HUPTI was the eighth proton center built in the U.S.

My Current Health Status

Prior to treatment, my PSA was 8.0 and my Gleason score was 3+2=5 from one pathology lab and 3+3=6 from another. There was no palpable tumor by DRE, so my cancer stage was labeled T1c. I was 57 years old.

Following treatment, my PSA dropped to below 1.0 and remained low ever since. To put this in perspective, prior to treatment, I never had a PSA reading below 3.5.

As I write this second edition of my book, it's more than 19 years since my treatment and the quality of my life couldn't be better. I'm experiencing no side effects whatsoever, and all my "plumbing" works just fine. If anything, my health and physical condition are better than before treatment.

My wife and I have continued an exercise regimen that was heavily influenced by our time at the Drayson Center. And, while our diet isn't perfect, it's quite healthful, having been influenced by our LLUCC experience and ongoing research.

There's no question that the Seventh-day Adventist diet and lifestyle – which we learned about while I was in treatment – promote good health and longevity. Adventists live as much as 10 years longer than the rest of us, and they are generally much healthier years.

A study funded by the U.S. National Institute on aging reported on this in the November 2005 issue of *National Geographic* Magazine. This was also documented in a book, *The Blue Zones: Lessons for Living Longer from the People Who've Lived the Longest.* The Adventist diet, largely a whole food, plant-based diet, is considered one of the most healthful diets in the world.

Our monthly *BOB Tales* newsletter has a section on health and we frequently include articles on foods for healthy living as well as foods that help prevent cancers of all types.

My diet is very low in animal fats, processed meats and red meats, as well as dairy products. I regularly drink almond milk, soymilk and pomegranate juice; I've increased the number of daily servings of fresh fruits and vegetables, including veggie and fruit "smoothies" for lunch most days during the week. And I've increased my daily intake of water.

I exercise six days a week. I was slightly overweight prior to treatment. Though diet and exercise, I've lost about 15 pounds, and am close to my ideal weight.

I take daily vitamins and supplements to support my health. More on diet and exercise later in this book, including, what I consider to be the best exercise in the world for good health.

CHAPTER 12

The Brotherhood of the Balloon

"Sometimes the most scenic roads in life are the detours you didn't mean to take."

– Angela Blount, Once Upon an Ever After

A Simple Beginning

Toward the end of treatment, my five new friends and I agreed that we'd stay in touch in order to continue our friendship and share information about our post-treatment journey. We would form an informal and private "proton men's club." I prepared a memo on my laptop computer in my rented apartment to document this special occasion. I jokingly addressed the memo to "The Brotherhood of the Balloon" reflecting the one thing we all had in common – the "gift" of a daily balloon, filled with water to protect our rectum during treatment and immobilize our prostate during beam delivery. Included in the memo was a form requesting contact information and cancer staging.

Members of this new fraternity willingly provided their information, returned the form to me, and the *Brotherhood of the Balloon* was born. Little did I know at the time what was to follow.

I had unknowingly left a couple of extra copies of the memo and sign-up sheet in the patient waiting room. And to my surprise, the next morning we had three new members, with a request for more memo-forms from the receptionist.

Following is the memo I sent to my five friends:

MEMO

TO: The Brotherhood of the Balloon ("BOB")

FROM: Bob Marckini

DATE: December 15, 2000

SUBJECT: Sharing Information

      I have spoken to a few of the guys who were treated in the October-December 2000 timeframe about keeping in touch in the coming months and perhaps years. Seeing that we all have something in common, it seems to make sense that we stay in touch and share information about our progress.

      My thinking is that we could share information on our PSAs, side effects, etc. We could make ourselves available to each other to discuss problems or questions that might arise. We could also perhaps make ourselves available to other guys with prostate cancer who are dealing with the trauma and challenges we experienced when we were diagnosed not so long ago.

      I suggest we use email as the primary vehicle for communication; however, if we all have each other's telephone number we can use the phone as well.

      I'll volunteer to collect, summarize, and forward any information you send to me.

      If you're interested in participating in this communication process, please provide the information requested below and return it to me before I leave on December 22nd, or provide it via email, phone, or regular mail. If you don't know some of the information, or do not wish to include it, just provide whatever information you're willing to share with the group. Thank you and good luck.

Name: _____   Email: _____

Address: _____

Phone: _____   Treatment end date: _____

Age: _____   Pretreatment PSA: _____

Gleason Score: _____   T- Score: _____

If you have any other suggestions for this communications process, please let me know.

When Gerry Troy and Dr. Lynn Martell heard about our "little group," they immediately saw something that I wouldn't see for some time. They recognized that something important was happening. This group that was forming could fill an important void in the lives of patients after treatment ended. It's human nature to go back to your "normal" routine when you return home. This might include a lifestyle characterized by poor diet, minimal exercise and no communication with men with whom you've just shared a life-changing experience. If former patients could keep in touch with each other, share information and support each other in the weeks, months and years ahead, then everybody wins.

According to the American Cancer Society: "Research has shown that being part of a support group following cancer treatment improves quality of life and enhances patient survival." Gerry and Lynn knew this; and they knew that patients who joined our group would benefit greatly from participation.

Tip: Being part of a support group after cancer treatment may not be "the manly" thing to do, but according to experts, it's good for your health and healing.

As a result, and unbeknownst to me, Gerry and Lynn became our marketing agents, talking-up the BOB at every opportunity.

At a patient Christmas party on the Monday before I left, Gerry announced to all in attendance that I had formed a new support group, and anyone interested in joining should see me.

The response surprised me. A few days later, when my wife and I left for home, we had 19 members of the *BOB*. I remember saying to my wife on the plane, "This was intended to be a small, private group of guys who just wanted to keep in touch – I suppose a few more won't matter. After all, the more, the merrier! But how can I possibly coordinate communications between 19 men from different parts of the country?"

A Life of Its Own

The word continued to spread at LLUCC after we left for home, mostly thanks to Gerry Troy and Dr. Lynn Martell. More and more patients wanted to join *The Brotherhood of the Balloon*. Each month Gerry would send me an envelope with a stack of sign-up sheets filled out by patients I had never met. Now I was beginning to feel pressure to turn this thing into something other than a small, "secret men's club."

Within weeks I was receiving phone calls from former patients who had heard of our organization and wanted to join. I began mailing out sign-up sheets from home and taking down member information over the phone.

The Brotherhood of the Balloon ("BOB") was taking on a life of its own. By December of 2001, our membership had grown to 282. Year-end 2002 saw membership at 736.

The best kept secret in medicine – proton therapy – was beginning to get out, much of this due to the efforts of our group to spread the word in our local communities on this exciting technology. As a result, more and more men were choosing proton therapy for their prostate cancer.

Members from Other Proton Centers

As new proton centers were built and opened, I began receiving requests from patients treated at these new centers to join our group, and I gladly accepted them. The more the merrier!

Today the *Brotherhood of the Balloon* has about 10,000 members from all corners of the earth – 50 U.S. states and 39 countries! There seems to be no end to our growth.

We have members in Germany, Puerto Rico, Singapore, Australia, Great Britain, Ecuador, Guam, Saipan, Palau, China, Canada, Italy, the Bahamas, the Philippines, Venezuela, and dozens of other locales. And members come from all walks of life including farmers, business leaders, physicians, scientists, educators, media personalities, professional athletes, clergy, engineers, bankers, lawyers, commercial pilots, stockbrokers, sports celebrities, ambassadors, and judges.

Our Mission

Initially our mission was simply to keep in touch and share information on how each of us was doing, weeks and months after treatment. As we grew, a real mission began to materialize.

Somewhere along the way, each of us began to realize that we were incredibly blessed to be among a tiny group of men who had received the "gift" of proton beam therapy for our prostate cancer. Our friends, family members and acquaintances with prostate cancer had chosen other options and so many of them had suffered the side effects of impotence, incontinence and even worse. We began to feel that we had an obligation to learn all we could about the technology that healed us; to tell the world about proton therapy; and to find a way to express our thanks and appreciation to the institution that treated us.

About two years into our existence, we formalized our three-part mission statement:

1. Provide a forum for aftercare support, communications and education;
2. Help others discover proton therapy;
3. Give something back to the institution that provided us with proton therapy

Newsletter

Since the beginning, the *BOB Tales* newsletter has been our primary communications vehicle with members. We started publishing the monthly newsletter in early 2001 and haven't missed an issue since. At the beginning, I remember wondering if I'd be able to find enough relevant and substantive material to fill a newsletter on a monthly basis. As it turns out, each month we have three or four times as much information as we can fit into each publication.

Every month we report on member feedback, prostate cancer prevention, detection, and treatment developments, BOB member reunions, new proton center announcements, how we're doing on our mission objectives, health and nutrition information, a brain teaser or riddle, and some humor to brighten the day.

Originally, we sent our newsletter out through my personal email system. As we grew larger, we overloaded that system and transitioned to a major email marketing firm to distribute our newsletter. This firm, which boasts more than one million clients, told us on more than one occasion that, of all their clients, we have the highest open and click-through rates – by a wide margin. That tells us our members are interested and they are engaged. It also tells us we must be doing something right with our newsletter content and reporting. We've also learned that many of our members forward copies of our newsletters to family members, friends and acquaintances. So, we are reaching lots of people with our communications.

Something in Common

When I was conducting my due diligence to find the best treatment option, I found that speaking with former patients – i.e. the "customers" – taught me far more about the various treatment options than all the books and articles I read, or the doctor interviews I conducted.

In designing the BOB application form, I made sure I captured enough information to be helpful to others in the future. I learned that not only do men like to talk with others of similar cancer stage, they often want to talk with someone of comparable age, profession, and sometimes even location.

Lawyers seem to like to talk with lawyers, clergy with clergy, physicians with physicians, and so on.

Dealing with prostate cancer all day can be a bit of a downer. So, I try to lighten things up now and then when talking with recently diagnosed men. One day, when I was in a giddy mood, I received a call from a gentleman who identified himself as a pilot. At that time, we had upwards of 50 pilots in our group, so I thought I'd have some fun with him:

"Would you like to speak with another pilot?" I asked.
"I'd love to," He replied.
"OK. Commercial or private?"
"Ah . . . private."
"Fixed wing or helicopter?"
"Are you serious? . . . uh, fixed wing."

"Piston engine or jet?"

"This is amazing," he said, "Piston."

"Single engine or twin?" I asked.

"Twin," he gasped. I could almost hear his jaw drop.

So, I gave him the name of one of our members who flies a twin-engine piston plane.

Flooded with Inquiries – Newly Diagnosed Men

As the word got out, through our membership and later our website, that I had done extensive research into the treatment options, I began receiving phone calls and emails from men who were diagnosed with prostate cancer. I gave willingly of my time, as I was once there myself, and others gave to me. Every day, I receive calls and emails, and they all start out pretty much the same way. "My name is 'Charlie,' I'm 59 years old and I've been diagnosed with prostate cancer. My PSA is . . . and my Gleason score is . . . "

I admit to being biased in favor of proton treatment. Many of the men I counsel choose the proton option, not so much because I'm "selling" them on it, but because of my passion for the technology that comes through in our conversations. The extensive data now available proves that this non-invasive treatment works. It does so without pain, anesthesia, catheters, and many of the risks associated with the other options; and add to this, many fewer side effects and complications than the alternatives.

When people call or email me, I just tell my story. I relate how important I feel it is to talk directly with patients who've chosen each of the options to learn firsthand about the treatment experience as well as life after treatment.

I direct them to our website and encourage them to read the FAQs, the member testimonials, and the studies and surveys posted there. Finally, I share with them what I learned during my own due diligence about the major treatment options, including the pros and cons of each.

I continue to learn more every day as our 10,000 members share with us the latest articles and information they find on prostate cancer prevention, diagnosis and treatment.

About a year after I completed my treatment, a businessman from Rhode Island called me after he had decided to have IMRT in

Florida. He had heard through a friend that I received proton therapy and was very happy with the results. We spoke several times. I shared the results of my research with him and put him in touch with the people at LLUCC. He flew out to the West Coast in his own plane and met with some of the medical staff. A week later he called to tell me he canceled his IMRT appointment and scheduled proton treatment in California. We have since become good friends. He's doing very well to this day and has recommended proton therapy to many friends and acquaintances.

Over the past 18 years I've spoken with literally thousands of people about my treatment – including a well-known psychologist from Massachusetts, a pilot from Montana, a dentist from Tennessee, a developer from Minnesota, a venture capitalist from Connecticut, a foreign ambassador, a business owner in London, a pastor in Hong Kong, a radio personality from Texas and hundreds more. Most have chosen the proton option, with very satisfactory results. Many of these men have become good friends.

There's a large and growing fraternity of prostate cancer survivors who are proton "graduates." There is a special bond between us. And for some reason this is much different from the relationships former patients have within other treatment modalities. Is it the protons? I'm not sure. But I do know there is something special in that connection, and it works to the benefit of us proton graduates.

Largest Organization of its Type in the World

Speaking of our large and growing fraternity. I have been told by leadership at the National Association for Proton Therapy (NAPT) that our group, *The Brotherhood of the Balloon*, is the largest group of patients in the world, who represent and promote a specific treatment modality. Our 10,000 members who have chosen proton therapy are staying connected and are keeping informed about the latest developments in proton therapy technology. They're also promoting proton therapy in their communities using a comprehensive PowerPoint presentation we provide; and they're making a difference.

One individual I spoke with a few years ago told me, "I chose proton therapy for my prostate cancer because it was the only treatment option with a fan club!" I thought about this and he's right. You could hardly expect thousands of former surgery patients to band together to promote radical prostatectomies for prostate cancer.

"I chose proton therapy for my prostate cancer, because it's the only treatment option with a fan club!"

Some Sad Cases

Unfortunately, in my communications with people on prostate cancer diagnosis and treatment, I've come across some sad cases. These usually had to do with individuals who, for various reasons, failed to have annual physical examinations, or had doctors who didn't believe in running routine PSA tests, or – believe it or not – had doctors who failed to recognize or respond to rapidly rising PSA.

One instance happened in May of 2002. The wife of a recently diagnosed prostate cancer patient called. She was doing research on treatment options for her husband and wanted to learn all she could about proton treatment from me.

After reminding her that I was not a physician and therefore could not give medical advice, only my opinion, I asked my typical opening questions: What is your husband's age, his PSA, his Gleason score, and is there a palpable tumor by DRE?

She told me he was 56 years old; his PSA was 37, his Gleason score was 10; and he had large tumors in both lobes of his prostate. My "knee-jerk" reaction was, "Surely this must have shown up in previous physical exams?" And she replied, "He's never had any physical exams. We don't believe in them. We prefer health food, meditation and yoga to conventional western medicine."

"Then how did you discover his cancer?" I asked. She replied, "He couldn't urinate, so we went to the hospital emergency room where they discovered the tumors."

What is so sad about this case is her husband was a young man. Routine physical examinations and blood tests would have detected his cancer years before. At this stage, it appeared to be too late. I wanted to tell her that the best advice I could offer was to have her husband get his affairs in order and prepare for the worst. But instead I told her I wasn't qualified to offer any suggestions in this case; I gave her the names of two physicians; and suggested she discuss her husband's case with them.

Another gentleman I spoke with seemed to be doing everything right – healthy diet, exercise and annual physical exams, including PSA screening. Sadly, his doctor didn't alert him to a problem until his PSA reached 61. It was then he discovered he had aggressive Gleason 10 prostate cancer. Fortunately for him, proton therapy solved his problem. His story is in the appendix.

Little did I know back on Aug. 10, 2000, when I received the call in Nantucket notifying me of my diagnosis, that years later I would be leading an international support group and counseling men all over the world. It's been an exciting and rewarding journey.

Our Mission

As mentioned above, our mission as a support group evolved over time into three objectives: 1) To provide aftercare support, communications and education to members, 2) To help others discover proton therapy by promoting it within our communities and beyond, and 3) To give back by encouraging financial contributions to proton therapy research. In the 19 years since our founding, we have done well in all three areas.

Aftercare support, communications and education happens through our formal communications (monthly newsletters) and informal communications (reunions, emails, and telephone). Numerous special educational projects have been initiated to aid individuals with specific questions or problems. Members without computers and email access are mailed hard copies of our newsletters.

We help others discover proton therapy through the special PowerPoint presentations we've prepared for our members. Our members deliver these presentations at community meetings, men's clubs, Lions Clubs, Rotary Clubs, support groups and church meetings.

We encourage members to write articles for their local newspapers as well as letters to the editor in national newspapers and magazines. Members also reach out to recently diagnosed men in one-on-one conversations. Each year, our group refers hundreds of men to

168

proton therapy – men who would otherwise have chosen surgery, seeds or some other treatment option.

Our giving-back efforts have also been remarkable. At a BOB member reunion in Washington state in 2004, one of our members proposed the establishment of the *Dr. James M. Slater Endowed Chair for Proton Therapy Research* at Loma Linda University Cancer Center. This was accepted, and our group funded the chair over the next few years to greater than $5 million.

Through our newsletters, we encourage our members to give back either directly or through their estate plan and members have been extremely generous in their response. An informal survey about 10 years ago showed that 40 percent of our members had made gifts for proton therapy research.

Giving Back – Marckini Endowed Chair and Other Ways

In June 2013, I was greatly honored to be invited to a Loma Linda University Health board meeting where BOB member Chuck Kubicki, a real estate developer from Cincinnati and now a close friend, announced the establishment of the *Robert J. Marckini Endowed Chair for Proton Research*. Mr. Kubicki "seeded" the new chair with a generous contribution.

Over the years, Chuck would make several more gifts to proton research. When LLUH announced their Vision 2020 campaign in 2015, Chuck made a $1 million gift.

To date, our group has made gifts totaling $13 million, mostly for proton therapy research and the *Robert J. Marckini Endowed Chair for Proton Therapy Research* is currently funded at approx.-imately $3 million.

Overall, it appears we're doing a pretty good job executing our mission.

Feedback

Emails and letters come in every day from both men and their wives, or significant others, who have benefited from our services, whether it be our website, our reference call lists, our one-on-one interactions, or my book. Here's one example:

I'm going for broke. I cancelled my surgery today . . . Last night I spoke at length with a BOB member who called me and was kind enough to spend time discussing his experiences and insights. It was a really great and uplifting conversation. Everyone in the Brotherhood I've corresponded with has been exceptionally helpful and encouraging. I'm sure you've heard this from others in my shoes, but you guys are lifesavers. I can't tell you adequately just how much the support and encouragement offered by the Brotherhood means after all the "doom and gloom" I previously encountered. With a bit of luck, I'll also be able to have the experience you all talk about, join the Brotherhood, and after a cure, help those who are just starting on their journey. My heartfelt thanks.

A New Website - www.protonbob.com

By early 2002, membership was growing at more than 30 new registrations per month, and our "manual" database, containing 22 pieces of information on more than 300 members was becoming impossible to manage.

I engaged my son-in-law's graphic design firm, Markus Design Group, to create a logo and establish a website for the BOB. The logo was perfect.

Next, they developed a website that went far beyond my expectations in terms of layout, attractiveness, features, and ease of navigation. In addition to the standard Home Page, Frequently Asked Questions (FAQs), About Us, Privacy Statements, Helpful Links, and other standard features, they provided some unique and user-friendly features. Here's our logo:

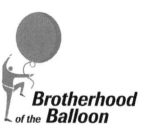

Password Protected

The site is split into two sections, one accessible to the general public, and the other password protected for members only. Prospective BOB members must be current or former proton patients or individuals who are scheduled for proton therapy for their prostate cancer. To become members, they visit our website home page, click on "Sign up," and provide their data, including their selected username and password.

Member List

All legitimate applications are accepted. Member information is stored on a comprehensive, member database. Name, address, email, phone numbers, age when treated, pretreatment PSA, Gleason score, T-stage, specific treatment received, current PSA, occupation, medical insurance carrier, and more are all displayed in one database. At this writing, there are about 220,000 pieces of data in our member database.

Newsletter

The secure part of the website also contains our monthly newsletter, *BOB Tales*. The newsletter is located in the secure area because members' names and some personal information are included in these publications.

Proton Patient Testimonials.

Member testimonials are the heart of our website. When I look back on what most influenced my treatment decision, it was talking with the "customers," the patients representing each treatment modality. Their stories meant so much to me; *it was the single most important factor in my decision.* For this reason, I decided to ask some of our members to document their journeys for our website. Today there are more than 100 testimonials on www.protonbob.com.

This has turned out to be the most important link on our website, in my opinion. On dozens of occasions, we've heard recently diagnosed men say they chose proton therapy largely as a result of reading these testimonials.

There are testimonials written by men from all walks of life, including Warren Johns, an attorney who happened to be consulting to the Loma Linda University Medical Center Board when they were considering making the huge capital investment for the proton facility. He voted against it at the time. Later, when he was diagnosed with prostate cancer, Warren became a beneficiary of proton therapy at Loma Linda's Cancer Center. Today, 25 years later, Warren is cancer free thanks to the healing power of the proton beam. He's now a strong proponent of proton therapy for prostate cancer and a member of our group.

Lots of physicians seem to gravitate to proton treatment. This alone is testimony to the efficacy of the technology.

Dr. Arnd Hallmeyer from Berlin, Germany, had a PSA of 436 when diagnosed in 2000. While working as a nurse in his early medical career, Dr. Hallmeyer assisted in performing radical prostatectomies. The invasiveness of those surgeries left an indelibly etched memory, which many years later, prompted him to search for a better alternative when diagnosed with prostate cancer. Today, he is cancer free and is a strong proponent for proton therapy.

Dr. Terry Wepsic's testimony is compelling. Dr. Wepsic's situation is unique. Not only is he a physician, he's a pathologist, cancer researcher and professor of pathology. When people with credentials like his choose proton therapy, others sit up and take notice.

During his consult with Dr. Rossi at LLUCC in early 2003, Terry looked at the doctor, and said, "I know you from somewhere." Dr. Rossi smiled and responded, "That's right. You were my pathology professor at Loyola."

Bob Reimer's testimonial is significant. Bob's PSA started rising rapidly in 1997. After ruling out infection, he was diagnosed with advanced prostate cancer, with PSA 61 and Gleason score 10. It doesn't get much worse than that. His doctor told him he probably had one to three years to live and he should go home, get his affairs in order, and prepare to die. That was more than 20 years ago. Bob discovered proton treatment. Today his PSA is 0.4; he's cancer free and has experienced no side effects.

Bill Hansell was a county commissioner in the state of Oregon. I met him while he and I were both in treatment at Loma Linda in 2000. I was impressed with his willingness to share his story with his community back home in Athena. He was writing weekly articles for his local newspaper, chronicling his prostate cancer journey and proton treatment experience. He also wrote a testimony for our website which has influenced many to choose proton therapy. Bill's journey has had an interesting recent development.

In 2012, Bill ran for and was elected state senator for the 29th District in Oregon. In 2019, he learned that constituents within his district and throughout the state of Oregon were being denied insurance coverage for proton therapy by their private insurers. This troubled him deeply, so he did something about it. He introduced legislation that would require insurers in the state of Oregon to cover proton therapy. Working behind the scenes with the insurance lobby and with colleagues on both sides of the aisle, he managed to get the bill passed – unanimously. Today, private insurers in Oregon are required to cover proton therapy to the same degree they cover other radiation treatment options. A big win.

Our members range in age from early 40s to late 90s. For many years, the senior citizen of our group was Charlie Einsiedler from Rhode Island. His story, on our website, is testimony to his engineering background, his tenacity, and his perseverance. He did considerable research when he was diagnosed at age 87, which included visiting premier medical institutions. And when his urologist suggested hormone therapy, Charlie refused because, "I'm too young for chemical castration," he said. Charlie lived 15 more years, free of cancer and side effects, and passed away at the age of 102 of natural causes. I remember talking with Charlie six years after his treatment at age 93. At that time, he was still playing golf three times a week. "I'm a bit frustrated," he admitted to me. "I find myself getting a bit tired after 18 holes."

Three of the testimonials on our website were written by former surgery patients who had a prostate cancer recurrence. They are Charlie Rubin, David Leighton and Bob Young. Their stories are compelling and are a chilling reminder that removing the cancerous gland from your body is not a guarantee of a cure. In fact, while I was at Loma Linda, I learned that about 5 percent of prostate cancer patients treated are former radical prostatectomy patients whose cancer returned after surgery.

All 100-plus testimonials provide value and insight to recently diagnosed men; they've been instrumental in leading hundreds – and maybe thousands – to proton therapy.

Help from the Institution that Saved My Life

I began the BOB organization covering all the expenses myself. As time went on the size and expenses grew exponentially. After a few years, I was giving some thought to shutting down the BOB and mentioned this to my friend, Dr. Lynn Martell at Loma Linda. Lynn had witnessed firsthand the value our group brought to newly diagnosed men as well as those in treatment and those post-treatment.

He also saw how effectively we were spreading the word about proton therapy around the world. He didn't want to see that stop. So, he offered to provide us with some financial support to help defray some of our expenses. This offer came with no strings attached: Membership in our group was not limited to Loma Linda patients. We were free to support newly diagnosed men who had chosen to be treated at other proton centers and to promote proton therapy worldwide.

We were back on track promoting prostate cancer awareness, prevention, proton therapy and pursuing our mission.

National Attention Through NBC Today Show

In early 2008 I received an email from NBC TV news journalist, George Lewis; he had recently been diagnosed with prostate cancer. George had done his homework, read my book, explored our website and was interested in proton therapy.

What an honor it was to hear from this man! Lewis – now retired – was a highly respected, senior news correspondent at NBC; winner of three Emmys as well as the George Foster Peabody award and the Edward R. Murrow award. Over the years I had watched him cover the Iraq war, Desert Storm, the Iran hostage crisis, revolutions in Romania, Latin American and Asia, the Tiananmen Square revolt in China, the OJ Simpson trial, the Exxon Valdez oil spill, fires in California and the Vietnam War. George was no stranger to crises.

We exchanged multiple emails and spoke by phone several times. George decided on proton treatment at Loma Linda and had a wonderful experience.

A few weeks after his treatment ended, he called and told me he was planning to do a segment for the Today Show and NBC Nightly News on his prostate cancer journey. He asked if he could bring his producer and a camera crew to my home in Massachusetts for part of the segment. I said, "Absolutely!"

George and the crew showed up a few days later, shooting several scenes, including one of him interviewing me in our back yard. Neighbors were lined up – outside of camera range – to observe the exciting event happening in our small community.

The piece aired a few weeks later and brought a lot of national attention to prostate cancer awareness and to proton therapy. The segment can be viewed on our website, www.protonbob.com.

Bringing in a Secret Weapon – Deb to the Rescue

In 2009, we were at 3,735 members in 50 states and 26 countries. We were adding about 50 new members each month. Newly diagnosed men and their spouses (or significant others) had learned about proton therapy, visited our website and wanted to learn more about this treatment option.

I was receiving about 40 email inquiries a day and spending several hours a day on the phone with them – seven days a week. Finding time to research and write a monthly newsletter, eat a few meals and get some sleep was becoming a real challenge. I needed help. *Badly.*

At the time, my daughter, Deb Hickey, was director of marketing for a successful search engine marketing firm. The company had outgrown their headquarters in a Boston suburb near Deb's home and was planning a move to a new location in downtown Boston. This represented a long commute through rush-hour traffic for Deb, something she wasn't looking forward to. She and her husband Mark were also in the process of adopting a baby.

Then the idea struck me. Deb was smart; she graduated from college with degrees in psychology and graphic design. Her writing, marketing and graphic-design skills were significant factors in the success of the firm she worked for. She had a warmth and magnetism that drew people to her; she had a sense of humor and great communication skills. And she was a person of faith. Deb was also a great listener and had a strong desire to help people. This was exactly the skillset I needed. And the bonus was that I'd have a chance to spend a lot of time with her.

But I thought, she doesn't know anything about prostate cancer or proton therapy. And she's a woman! But I knew nothing about prostate cancer or proton therapy when I was diagnosed, and years later I've written two books on the subject. Also, almost half the people I talk with are women – spouses, significant others, sisters, daughters, and even mothers of recently diagnosed men. It was the skills that Deb could bring to the table that could be so helpful to me and our mission.

So, I approached her. And her first reaction was, "Are you serious?" But after much discussion, and all the salesmanship, charm, coercion and persuasion skills I could muster, Deb agreed to give it a try.

I quickly learned that Deb brought far more to the table than I ever could have imagined. She was a quick study on the technology of proton therapy; and her administrative and IT skills were exactly what I needed. One by one, she fixed all our broken and outdated systems, redesigned the patient-registration form, rebuilt our website, and completely revamped our newsletter format, style and distribution system.

Today, Deb has taken over most of the responsibilities of running the BOB organization. She manages our website, Facebook page and blog. She researches the stories and writes most of our monthly newsletter. She represents us at the National Association for Proton Therapy (NAPT) as a participant and speaker. She's a team member in the COMPPARE trial organization. And she's a patient advocate representative on the Proton Therapy Law Coalition, working with law firms, proton centers, and other advocates to reverse the trend of denials by private insurers for proton therapy. Our members love her and newly diagnosed patients who reach her through our website find a knowledgeable, sensitive and compassionate resource.

176

Most importantly, Deb's given her ol' man an opportunity to take some time off, travel, and play some golf.

In all humility, I must admit it was a brilliant move on my part to bring Deb into the organization!

Transfer of BOB Ownership

Our organization continued to grow in size, complexity . . . and workload. Our systems were getting tired, outdated and in need of serious upgrade. We no longer had the resources and expertise to deal with the administrative, IT and legal issues that accompany an institution of the size ours had grown. Coincidentally I was spending more and more time working on the second edition of my book and, also began to move toward retirement ... for the third time. After talking with my friends at Loma Linda, at my request, we transferred ownership of the Brotherhood of the Balloon to Loma Linda University Health (LLUH).

The folks at LLUH were receptive to this idea, fundamentally because it ensured continuity of our ministry and the work we were doing promoting prostate cancer awareness, education and proton therapy.

The good news is, we gained access to LLUH's vast professional resources without having to change direction. We continue to register members treated at proton centers in the U.S., Europe and Asia. And LLUH has made no demands on us, other than asking that we respect federal law on patient health information confidentiality, as well as the organization's mission and values.

Their support has been phenomenal; we've continued to advance our mission; grow our membership, educate men and their loved ones on prostate cancer awareness, prevention and treatment; and promote the benefits of proton therapy.

And thank God for Deb's growing involvement and leadership. She now runs just about all BOB operations while her dad settles back.

"It's a wonderful life."

CHAPTER 13

The Medical Insurance Challenge

This subject is so important I felt a chapter should be devoted to it.

"You may never know what results come from your action. But if you do nothing, there will be no result."
— *Mahatma Gandhi*

One More Difference Between Procedures

As you've read in this book, there are many differences between prostate cancer treatment options. But there's one more important difference between proton treatment and all the other options – cost.

Cost of Surgery

Radical prostatectomies are performed in operating rooms. These are the same operating rooms that are used for appendectomies, tonsillectomies, heart bypasses, hernia repairs, and the like. In other words, these procedures are carried out in conventional hospital operating rooms that can be used for limitless surgical procedures.

Specialized equipment required for these procedures generally costs from tens of thousands to a few hundred thousand dollars and can be brought into the operating room.

A radical prostatectomy requires a surgeon, anesthesiologist, pathologist, surgical assistants, and follow-up care by nursing staff and physicians during the short hospital stay. Subsequent visits for catheter management and removal and consults are also part of the radical prostatectomy process.

All this costs money. But, once again, the procedure is done in a conventional operating room, and the cost of this facility is shared by many of the other procedures performed there. Likewise, the recovery room, the hospital room, the nursing staff, etc. are all shared by a large patient population and a wide variety of medical procedures, all helping to keep the cost of these procedures down.

So, if a radical prostatectomy costs the medical insurer $25,000 (or even $35,000 to $40,000 at the pricier centers of excellence), generally speaking, everybody is happy. The doctor and hospital earn a profit, as they should; the insurance company pays a reasonable amount for the procedure; and the patient pays nothing, or perhaps a small deductible on his policy.

Cost of the Other Treatment Options

Most of the other procedures are performed in similar facilities, with staffs that handle numerous other medical procedures.

Most forms of external beam radiation are done in conventional radiotherapy treatment facilities. Certain specialized devices are used to focus the beam and/or modulate radiation energy. In the case of IMRT, for example, the price tag for specialized equipment is reported to be in the $1 million range. Again, this procedure is done in a conventional hospital setting, with staff that handles many other medical procedures and tasks.

In the case of conventional (X-ray) three-dimensional conformal radiation, patient work up and preparation (imaging, studies, interdisciplinary consultations, etc.) are similar, and thus costs for this portion of treatment are similar.

Brachytherapy and cryosurgery may require some specialized equipment and instrumentation as well, but these procedures also can be performed in a conventional setting.

The bottom line: Specialized equipment and capital costs for doing most of the aforementioned procedures are modest. Also, facilities, equipment, and personnel for these procedures are typically shared with other medical procedures. The costs, therefore, can be shared and thus maintained in a moderate range, allowing both hospital and physician to earn a profit and the insurer to pay a modest sum for the above procedures, reportedly in the $20,000 to $40,000 range per patient.

The situation with proton therapy is quite different.

Why Proton Therapy Costs More

Since inception, proton therapy has cost more, primarily because of the capital investment needed to build a proton treatment facility. More than $150 million is typically required to purchase the particle accelerator and build a facility with multiple hundred-ton rotating gantries and computer-control systems. They also require a number of people to operate and maintain these complex systems. Also, considerable real estate is needed to house the particle accelerator and multiple three-story-high concrete-and-steel treatment gantries.

A large staff is needed to manage the synchrotron or cyclotron during the treatment process and to do daily calibration and maintenance. Physicists and dosimetrists are required to plan and manage patient-customized treatment protocols. Add to that the dedicated oncologists, case managers, nurses, and radiation therapists, and the cost of staff becomes significant. Multi-treatment room proton treatment centers can require a staff of 80 or more people to operate.

As a result of all these factors, it costs more money to treat prostate cancer with proton therapy than with other treatment modalities.

What is the payoff for the patient? Very simply, it's quality of life. In some cases, it's life itself. Proton beam therapy has been shown to cure more than 45 cancers and other diseases, including some that are untreatable by other means. And in the case of prostate cancer, it can clearly be shown that there's less collateral damage to surrounding organs and tissue, and therefore side effects should be lower than with other options, short of active surveillance.

The Medicare system recognizes the value of proton therapy and since 1988 has willingly paid the higher price for this premium treatment.

The Superiority of Proton Therapy

The laws of physics, multiple patient surveys and anecdotal evidence points to the fact that proton therapy is superior to all forms of conventional X-ray treatment options. Certainly advanced IMRT technologies do a much better job than conventional/conformal X-ray modalities of the past, but they still use X-rays, which means everything in the path of the beam is radiated, both as the beam enters the body and as it leaves the body after passing through the tumor volume.

As mentioned previously, one thing doctors, physicists and other scientists agree on is that the only safe dose of radiation to healthy tissue is a zero dose. Proton therapy comes much closer to that goal than any advanced form of IMRT, which uses X-rays. That being the case, one can only conclude that the patient is better served with protons than with IMRT. Less radiation to heathy tissue means lower chance of damage to surrounding organs and tissues and significantly lower chances of secondary, radiation-induced cancers later in life.

But here's the problem: The long, complex and costly randomized clinical trials proving this have yet to be completed. As noted above, surveys and anecdotal evidence show proton's superiority. The laws of physics also predict the benefits of proton. But private insurers have learned that they can "get away" with denying coverage for more costly proton therapy because it has not been *proven scientifically* to be superior to lower cost IMRT.

A reasonable position to take? Not necessarily. Note that scientific studies were never conducted to prove that IMRT was superior to old fashioned conformal X-ray technology, but the insurers willingly pay for IMRT. Why? Because the cost is about the same. Sadly, it seems to be all about money with private insurers.

Fortunately, Medicare has consistently paid for prostate cancer proton therapy, so men over 65 with Medicare typically have no difficulty with coverage. The problem has been with private insurers. And that problem has become more and more of a challenge over time.

Appealing Denials Used to be Easy

Ten years ago, fighting denials for prostate cancer proton therapy was relatively easy. Back then, private insurers would typically deny claims based on proton therapy being "experimental" and/or "investigational."

Our organization, *The Brotherhood of the Balloon* assisted hundreds of men with their appeals on that specific denial. Our approach was simple. First, we disputed the "experimental" and/or "investigational" claim by noting that proton therapy has been used for treating cancer since the early 1950s and that well over 100,000 patients have been treated with proton therapy – mostly prostate cancer patients. Secondly, we pointed out that proton therapy was FDA approved in 1988. So, a medical treatment that was both FDA approved and used to treat more than 100,000 patients could hardly be considered "investigational" or "experimental."

And thirdly, when we sorted our extensive member database by insurance carriers, we could easily point out that XYZ insurance company had reimbursed patients treated with protons for prostate cancer dozens of times in the past. Case closed. Easy win! Or so it was in the past. Our member database was of enormous benefit with insurance denials back then.

We also put together an *Insurance Appeals Strategy Document* (ASD), which contains game plans and tactics for appealing denied insurance claims for proton therapy. The file contains information on FDA approval for proton therapy, a list of private insurers who have covered proton therapy in the past, and some form letters with arguments for most types of denial. The ASD has helped many newly diagnosed men win their appeals.

That's the good news. The bad news is that almost all private insurers have learned they can save money by denying coverage for proton therapy. They're digging in their heels and fighting harder than ever when the appeals come in.

Many newly diagnosed men have told me that it's bad enough to learn you have a life-threatening disease like prostate cancer. But to then go through the long and arduous process of studying the treatment alternatives, meeting with doctors, searching the Internet, interviewing former patients and then learn the treatment you have chosen will not be covered by your insurance is devastating.

Some are so sold on proton therapy they choose to pay out of pocket – sometimes tens of thousands of dollars – taking money from savings, IRAs or through home mortgages.

Many of the proton centers have hired staff to help patients with the appeals process. During the early stages of this process, most denials were overturned, and the patients were able to have their treatment. But, over time, the insurers fought harder, dug their heels in even deeper, and more and more patients lost their appeals. Today only a small percentage of patients with private insurance win their appeals. And this often requires much help from the proton center and/or assistance from an attorney (See information on the *Proton Therapy Law Coalition* below).

Sadly, many men tire of the battle, become frustrated with the process, grow anxious about their treatment delays and reluctantly choose IMRT, which their insurer will cover. I refer to this as "Denial by Delay," a practice that's been quite successful for private insurers who don't want to pay for the higher cost of proton therapy.

There's Reason for Hope with Insurance Coverage

At this writing, there are many factors at play, some of which will likely have favorable impact on private insurer coverage for prostate cancer proton therapy. I will describe a few.

1. Newer Single-room Proton Centers May Help Lower Cost

Several companies are building self-contained single-room proton treatment centers that cost considerably less than the original multi-gantry treatment centers. One such system costs about $40 million.

The advantage of these lower-cost, single-room systems is that the price to enter this previously exclusive technological market is more affordable to a larger number of medical centers. Lower capital costs, smaller staffs and operating at, or near, capacity allows these centers to function at lower costs than traditional, large proton centers. Eventually this should lead to lower treatment cost. Once the

184

cost of proton therapy approaches the cost of IMRT, private insurers will become more "proton friendly" and denials will disappear.

2. Hypofractionation Technology

Because the proton beam can be so precisely delivered to the tumor volume, researchers have found they can significantly increase the dose per treatment (fraction) and deliver proton therapy over a smaller number of days/weeks. Essentially all proton centers in the U.S. and some in Europe and Asia are running trials on hypo-fractionation. Some, like MD Anderson, have made hypofractionation the standard treatment protocol for early- and mid-stage prostate cancer patients.

With hypofractionation, instead of 40 to 44 treatments, five days a week over eight to nine weeks for prostate cancer patients, proton centers are treating patients with higher doses in 20 to 24 treatments over four to five weeks. Extreme hypofractionation, using Stereotactic Body Radiation Therapy (SBRT), a five-treatment hypofractionation approach is also showing promise.

Higher doses and fewer treatments, translates into lower overall cost for treatment, theoretically approaching the cost of IMRT. If/when hypofractionation becomes a standard treatment protocol, and costs begin to approach IMRT levels, insurers will have no more reason to deny coverage.

I am optimistic that as this technology is optimized, a) the patient will benefit by having shorter treatment schedules, b) there will be no change in disease-free survival or quality of life, and c) the resulting lower cost will reduce or eliminate the barrier of private insurer coverage.

Trials continue at all proton centers. It is yet to be determined when this technology might be fully approved and adopted, or for what cancer stages it can be successfully used.

3. Clinical Trials Comparing Proton and IMRT

If a clinical trial comparing proton to IMRT – head-to-head – were to show that proton therapy is superior to IMRT as measured by either disease-free survival or quality of life (urinary, bowel, sexual function) after treatment, then insurers would literally be forced to pay for the more costly proton therapy.

But there have been formidable challenges with initiating clinical trials. These include:

- **Funding:** Clinical trials cost millions of dollars and securing funding of these trials is an enormous effort.

- **Accruing Patients:** A randomized clinical trial comparing proton to IMRT uses *chance* to divide people into the two groups. Patients cannot select which treatment they will receive. One such trial, funded a few years ago, has been extremely slow to get off the ground due to slow patient accrual. When patients learn of the differences between proton and IMRT – particularly regarding radiation exposure to healthy tissue – they often refuse to be randomized, as they prefer to be in the proton arm.

- **Time:** Even if funding can be secured and patients can be accrued, it takes months to design the study, one to two years to accrue the patients and about five years before meaningful data can be collected to prove any hypothesis.

Two Very Important Trials are Under Way

Despite the challenges of funding, patient accrual and time, there are two critically important trials that will help to answer the question, once and for all, about the relative value of proton therapy vs. IMRT.

PARTIQoL Trial: The acronym PARTIQoL stands for Prostate Advanced Radiation Technologies Investigating Quality of Life. The name is also a play on the term "particle therapy," which refers to the proton segment of the trial. This is a comprehensive, randomized clinical trial with a targeted 400 participants. The study is being funded by The National Cancer Institute (NCI) and Massachusetts General Hospital (MGH).

186

I spoke recently with Jason Efstathiou, M.D. Director of Genitourinary Services, Department of Radiation Oncology at MGH about the PARTIQoL trial. Dr. Efstathiou is the principal investigator on this important project. He told me that thirty-six institutions are involved in this study, 15 of which are main proton centers. He further reported that all 400 patients have been registered and that 50 more are being added.

The focus of the trial will be on patient- and physician-reported results two years after treatment and beyond. Some of the variables being studied include moderate hypofractionation, the use of rectal spacers, and pencil beam scanning.

In addition to biochemical control, endpoints in the study will include urinary, bowel, sexual function, and other quality-of-life issues. Initial treatment cost as well as follow-up treatment costs will also be monitored. Results of this trial are expected to be published in 2023.

Tom Pisansky, M.D. Mayo Clinic said, "The PARTIQoL Trial is a landmark and pioneering study that serves as a model for technology assessment."

COMPPARE Trial: This is the most recent study comparing proton therapy to IMRT for treating prostate cancer.

The study is being funded by PCORI (Patient Centered Outcome Research Institute) and is being called the COMPPARE, trial. The double Ps represent the collaborative effort by proton and photon practitioners, patients, stakeholders and PCORI to answer the important question of whether there are meaningful result differences between protons and photons for men with prostate cancer.

The study is being led by Nancy Mendenhall, MD, Medical Director at University of Florida Health Proton Therapy Institute.

Dr. Mendenhall has assembled an impressive team of physicians, scientists, statisticians, advisers and patients, and is vigorously driving this study toward a set of ambitious goals with an aggressive timetable. Dr. Mendenhall has said:

This is a critically important study that will compare outcomes between proton and conventional radiation in cohorts of 3,000 men with prostate cancer. It will determine whether there are differences in disease control, toxicity and quality of life in survivors – providing much-needed answers

187

to patients, families, medical teams, hospitals, insurers and policy makers.

Most proton therapy centers in the U.S. are participating as well as several IMRT centers. Deb Hickey and I are "stakeholders" on the study. Deb serves as a patient caregiver, and I serve on the executive board as well as on the patient stakeholder group.

To learn more about the COMPPARE Trial, visit: https://comppare.org.

4. NAPT and The Alliance for Proton Therapy Access

The National Association for Proton Therapy (NAPT: www.proton-therapy.org) and The Alliance for Proton Therapy Access (https://allianceforprotontherapy.org) are two critically important proton therapy support organizations that promote patient advocacy. Their efforts in fighting insurance denials and in other areas, have played a key role in helping to ensure that proton therapy is available to patients seeking advanced, precisely targeted radiotherapy for treating their cancers.

5. The Proton Therapy Law Coalition Initiative

On May 10, 2019, a group of 35 proton therapy providers, proton patient advocates, and attorneys convened for the first *Proton Therapy Legal Summit* held in Orange County, CA. Deb Hickey and I represented the BOB at the meeting as patient advocates.

The summit was hosted by two Southern California-based law firms, Kantor & Kantor, LLP (Northridge, CA) and Callahan & Blaine (Santa Ana, CA) who on March 26, 2019, filed a nationwide Employee Retirement Income Security Act (ERISA) class action lawsuit against UnitedHealthcare challenging its use of internally-developed clinical guidelines to justify widespread and systematic denials of proton therapy when such denials go against generally accepted standards of care.

The goal of the summit was to launch the formation of the Proton Therapy Law Coalition, an alliance devoted to bringing together proton therapy providers, patient-advocacy groups and skilled ERISA and bad-faith insurance litigation attorneys to collaborate on strategies to bring about nationwide pressure on insurance companies to cover proton therapy. The approach of the coalition is holistic, seeking to coordinate and maximize the collective skills of participating providers, advocates and attorneys during the claims and appeals process in courtrooms and in state legislative chambers.

The Challenge

On one side are the insurance companies, which are completely unified in denying coverage to patients ostensibly because proton therapy is "experimental," "investigational" or hasn't been proven through randomized clinical trials to be superior to IMRT, thus justifying the higher reimbursement cost.

On the other side, there's a divergence of focus and interests – academic and private proton therapy centers and advocacy groups strewn across the country, with newly diagnosed patients desperately seeking proton therapy to destroy their cancers. And what's been missing is a coordinated and unified effort to deal with the powerful insurance machine. Until now.

A Solution

Insurance companies will feel the weight of their wrongful denials of proton therapy only if it affects their bottom lines. And the only way to affect their bottom lines – under current conditions – is to force them to appear in courtrooms, spend money on civil defense attorneys and make them open their pocketbooks to settlements and judgments.

The two law firms represented in the summit have had recent success in fighting insurance companies over health claim denials. Participants in the summit thus agreed to:

- Reach out to proton therapy providers to gauge interest in having attorneys assist with insurance denials and the appeals process.

- Seek to work with interested providers in crafting coverage recommendations to major U.S. employers with self-funded health plans to persuade employers to cover proton therapy.
- Work with interested current and former patients who would like to enforce their legal rights in the claims/appeals process or in the courtroom where appropriate.
- Work toward the goal of getting model proton therapy access legislation in the hands of the National Conference of State Legislatures.
- Continue to reach out to providers and advocacy groups interested in working together to create real change.

We all agreed that we can't wait any longer. It's time to force the insurance companies to change their practices.

The Bottom Line

As of this writing, Medicare in the U.S. routinely covers proton therapy for prostate cancer while most private insurers have changed their policies and are denying reimbursement for higher-cost proton therapy.

Patients who are not yet on Medicare, who have done their homework and have learned of the advantages of proton therapy are not giving up. Many fight the denials through the appeals process and some win, often with help from the treating institution and/or legal counsel, but not without significant effort.

Some elect to pay out-of-pocket for proton therapy and choose to fight the denial after the fact. And sadly, some give up the fight and go with one of the options their insurance will cover.

The time is coming – soon, I expect – when the efforts described above will result in private insurers changing their policies and covering proton therapy for prostate cancer.

I hope to be reporting this happy development when I write the third edition of this book.

CHAPTER 14

What if My Treatment Fails?

"Ninety-nine percent of the things you worry about never happen."

– Peaceful Diaries

Fortunately, for most men with early- or mid-stage disease, this is not something you'd ever have to deal with. But it's worth talking about since it's a subject that's often on a patient's mind, particularly when deciding between treatment options.

For men who choose surgery as their primary treatment option, the most common salvage treatment following a localized recurrence is radiation therapy. If the recurrence, following surgery is not localized, i.e. is metastatic, then some form of systemic treatment is typically ordered.

What Does Treatment Failure Mean?

To properly deal with this subject one must first understand what the term "treatment failure" means. Before PSA was used as a relative prostate cancer marker, failure was determined by either prostate cancer symptoms (blood in the urine, pelvic pain, urinary tract problems, etc.) or by the presence of a lump in the prostate area detected by DRE. As mentioned in an earlier chapter, the term cNED (no Clinical Evidence of Disease) is used to describe this process.

Today, the PSA measurement has added a new dimension to monitoring a patient following prostate cancer treatment, regardless of the treatment chosen. The term bNED (no Biochemical Evidence of Disease) refers to post-treatment PSA behaving in a certain fashion.

PSA comes from two sources: 1) a functioning prostate (prostate tissue), or 2) prostate cancer. Therefore, if one chooses surgery and has the prostate removed, post-treatment PSA should be non-detectable, because the prostate has been removed. So, any measurable PSA would indicate the presence of prostate cancer after surgery.

For all other treatments, which leave the prostate in place – albeit "damaged" by the treatment process – one would expect to see low levels of PSA in the bloodstream. If the cancer has been destroyed, however, this PSA level, produced by the remaining prostate tissue, should be much lower than pretreatment levels and should be relatively stable. Multiple increases in PSA following external beam radiation therapy (proton or IMRT), brachytherapy, or cryosurgery, *could* be indicative of biochemical failure (see Phoenix definition earlier in this book), thus cancer activity. A single high reading should be no cause for alarm. PSA "bumps" are common after non-surgical treatments.

If there are multiple PSA increases, indicating the probability of cancer activity (biochemical failure), or if there is clinical failure as detected either by DRE or the presence of prostate cancer symptoms, all is not lost. This is *not* a death sentence.

"Biochemical or clinical failure is not a death sentence."

False Alarms

The first thing to do is to rule out false alarms. False alarms are much more common than cancer recurrences. Patients – and even some doctors – often jump to conclusions when there's a PSA bump (or two) after treatment. PSA bumps are quite common following radiotherapy and shouldn't be interpreted as a recurrence.

One of our members experienced a bump in his PSA. His local oncologist concluded that his cancer had returned and recommended he begin triple blockade hormonal therapy. The patient solicited a second opinion from another physician who recommended rechecking his PSA. The retest showed his PSA back in line. Today, many years after treatment, his PSA is holding steady at 0.3.

An article in the journal, *Urology* (62:683-688, 2003) reported on a study conducted on several men who had brachytherapy (seeds) for their prostate cancer. Eight of the men in the study saw their PSA initially decline, and then turn around. Each experienced three to five successive increases in PSA, all within 30 months of treatment. Biopsies on *every* one of these men showed cancer in the prostate. This is not uncommon during the first two to three years following radiotherapy. But here's the interesting part: In *all* eight cases, no action was taken; PSA turned around, began to decline, and settled down at nadirs of less than 1.0. Researchers concluded:

> *Transient PSA rises can occur even in the presence of a persistently positive biopsy, and patients and physicians should not feel compelled to rush ahead with salvage therapy. Based on patient data reported here, it appears that a temporary spike up to 10 ng/mL may still be consistent with cancer eradication.*

Some feel their PSA nadir following radiotherapy must be close to zero for them to be "cured." Not true. While doctors will tell you, "The lower the nadir the better," there are men who have been cured of prostate cancer whose PSAs showed nadirs above 1 or even 2.

The following discussion in this chapter is based on a confirmation of cancer recurrence.

"Some feel their PSA nadir following radiotherapy must be close to zero for them to be 'cured.' Not true!"

PSA Velocity

It's entirely possible, that the primary treatment destroyed (or removed) most, but not all the cancer. The remaining cancer cells, which would produce some PSA in the blood, may continue growing at a rate that is slow enough (indolent cancer) to be of no concern. This is especially true if the patient is elderly or has co-morbidities and is likely to die of other causes before the prostate cancer can begin to produce symptoms.

"The remaining cancer cells, which would produce some PSA in the blood, may continue growing at a rate that is slow enough (indolent cancer) to be of no concern."

Dr. Charles E. "Snuffy" Myers, medical oncologist, founder of the American Institute of Disease of the Prostate, and world-renowned prostate cancer expert, wrote an excellent article on this subject, referencing studies by R.S. Pruthi and C.R. Pound, both listed in the bibliography in the appendix.

First Steps

In the event the recurrent cancer is growing fast and action is needed, there are several steps that should be taken before any treatment decision is made. This could be the subject for another book but will be summarized here.

Typically, imaging tests can be conducted to determine the location of any cancer activity. As of this writing, 3-Tesla, multi-parametric MRI is leading-edge technology for finding suspicious lesions *within* the prostate.

Overlaying this imaging with ultrasound-guided biopsy (i.e. MRI fusion-guided biopsy) can help to stage any cancer that might be present in the prostate.

To look for cancer outside the prostate there are multiple tests available. A bone scan helps to identify any cancer in the skeletal system. New state-of-the-art PET/CT imaging techniques such as C-11 Choline, C-11 Acetate, Axumin and Gallium 68 PSMA help to find even the tiniest metastatic lesions throughout the body.

Depending on the results of these tests, any one of several salvage treatment options could be prescribed.

Salvage Options – Localized Recurrence

A slow PSA progression with long PSA doubling times may be an indication of a rather indolent (non-aggressive) cancer recurrence. In this case, it might be advisable for the patient to do nothing other than active surveillance, monitoring PSA periodically.

Patients with rapidly rising PSA following external beam radiation therapy (proton or IMRT) have several salvage options available to them if tests show the cancer is still contained within the prostate. These options include internal radiation (brachytherapy), targeted pencil beam proton therapy, cryosurgery, and salvage radical prostatectomy. The latter is more complicated than primary radical prostatectomy but is being done by specialists in major medical centers.

High Intensity Focused Ultrasound (HIFU) may also be an alternative, but this procedure is still relatively new and little data is available on HIFU for salvage.

Salvage Options – with Metastasis

When the recurrent cancer is determined to be *outside* the prostate, there are still many options available, including treatments with curative intent.

If imaging tests show five or fewer lesions, the cancer is said to be oligometastatic. This is a relatively new concept and with today's technology for imaging and treatment, patients with oligometastatic disease often have an excellent long-term prognosis.

Recurrent oligometastatic disease (five or fewer metastatic lesions) can often be treated with curative intent.

Depending on the location of the lesions, salvage treatment for oligometastatic patients can include pencil beam proton, IMRT surgery, cryotherapy, brachytherapy, HIFU, hormonal therapy, or some combination of these treatment options.

For more significant metastasis, systemic treatment is commonly prescribed by doctors. The most common systemic treatment is androgen deprivation therapy (ADT), also called Hormone Ablation Therapy (HAT) or hormonal therapy.

The male hormone, testosterone, is known to fuel prostate cancer growth. Hormonal therapy helps to reduce the amount and activity of testosterone, thus slowing the advancement of prostate cancer.

There are several agents that can be used, often in combination, the most common being Lupron, Casodex and Zoladex.

As mentioned earlier, Intermittent Hormonal Therapy (IHT) is more commonly used to treat advanced/metastatic prostate cancer. The benefit in using IHT is a reduction in the intensity of side effects, and for many, a longer period of disease control before the hormonal therapy loses its effectiveness. Hormonal therapy is generally not used with curative intent.

Another systemic treatment commonly used to treat advanced prostate cancer is chemotherapy. Chemotherapy drugs, such as Taxotere (docetaxel) or Jevtana (cabazitaxel) are commonly used when prostate cancer no longer responds to hormonal therapy.

Vaccine treatments are also employed to treat advanced prostate cancer. Provenge (sipuleucel-T) has been proven to prolong survival in many patients with hormone resistant disease.

Secondary Endocrine Therapy is also used to treat hormone-resistant cancer. Ketoconazole inhibits adrenal and testicular synthesis of testosterone. This drug is typically given with hydrocortisone to prevent adrenal insufficiency.

Research on vaccines that alter the body's immune system using genetically modified viruses are showing promise. One of these vaccines manipulates blood cells from the patient's own immune system causing them to attack the cancer.

Technology is advancing rapidly. Much of what I've reported here didn't exist when I was treated in 2000, or when I published the first edition of my book in 2006.

Recurrences Can Happen with All Treatment Options

No surgeon or radiation oncologist can guarantee that you'll be cured if you choose his/her treatment option. I learned this early on in my research. One reason proton therapy was so attractive to me is that, based on my research, the quality of my life would be best preserved with proton. And, if I were to have a recurrence 10 or 20 years later, it would give researchers 10 or 20 more years to develop better ways to detect, treat, and even cure recurrent prostate cancer. And the fact is, these exciting new technologies are emerging.

New imaging technologies can detect millimeter-sized lesions both within and outside the prostate. There are new internal and external treatment protocols, new medications, and new approaches to dealing with recurrent disease that didn't exist when I was diagnosed.

In Summary

My belief is that the prostate cancer patient should choose the treatment option that gives him the best chance of a cure along with the best expected quality of life after treatment. Biochemical failures can and will happen with some – but thankfully a small minority of patients. Mild recurrences – particularly in older men – can often be monitored with some form of active surveillance. For others, new technologies and medications are continually being developed that can offer patients several viable options for dealing with a recurrence. And these technological changes are happening at an accelerating pace.

CHAPTER 15

The Benefits of Proton Therapy

"The river of knowledge has no depth."
– Chinonye J. Chidolue

A whole book could be written on this subject. I'll try to limit my comments to information I've picked up on proton therapy since I published the first edition of my book 14 years ago.

As I've mentioned earlier, there are numerous and disparate options for treating localized prostate cancer. All have their pros and cons as well as their supporters and their detractors. Doctors and institutions that practice individual treatment modalities or even multiple modalities, predictably promote what they have to offer.

If a person walks into a Mercedes dealership and says, "I'm interested in buying a new car," you're not going to hear the store manager say, "There's a BMW dealership down the street; they have some great models on sale right now; why not go take a look."

For purposes of this chapter, I'll assume that I have your attention and that you are thinking seriously about choosing proton therapy for your prostate cancer.

Surveying Our Membership

In early 2009, the holding company that managed a major private insurer in four large states announced they would no longer be reimbursing for proton therapy for prostate cancer, lung cancer, esophageal cancer or hepatocellular carcinoma effective June 1, 2009. This prompted an angry response by our membership, which was then approaching 4,000, representing roughly half the men who had been treated with proton therapy for prostate cancer in the world at that time. We were deluged with emails and phone calls from members asking what they could do about it. We attempted letter writing campaigns, but these were largely ignored.

In April 2009, I decided to do an email survey of our membership to determine just how satisfied former prostate cancer patients were with their proton therapy decision, thinking that perhaps we could use this information to help reverse the tide of private insurers denying proton therapy coverage.

At that time, we had 2,913 members with working emails. Having conducted surveys in my professional life, I knew that, depending on the group surveyed a 10 - 15 percent response to a survey is considered average, and a 30 – 40 percent response was considered excellent. I was not prepared for what was to come.

On April 9, 2009, we sent the survey by email to 2,913 BOB members who had computers and email capability. We also asked sponsors to print out hard copies of the survey, send them to their "sponsorees," and ask them to mail the surveys to our data center in Englewood, CO.

Three weeks after the survey was sent out, we had heard from 1,520 members, representing 52 percent of our members with working emails, which was 39 percent of our total membership, and roughly 20 percent of the all men alive at that time, who had been treated with protons for prostate cancer – a phenomenal response!

Ninety-five percent of those who responded said proton therapy was their first treatment for prostate cancer. Five percent were former surgery patients who were treated with protons after a cancer recurrence.

In retrospect, I could have worded some questions differently to elicit more definitive information. For example, where I asked the question, "Have you experienced any problems or changes," many respondents checked, "Yes," and they reported changes that were totally unrelated to their proton therapy. And they even mentioned that fact. They just seemed compelled to report this for some reason. Nevertheless, I think we had what we needed for our purposes.

On April 22, 2009, we took a snapshot of the returns and prepared some charts and graphs. At that time, we had about 1,450 returns. The graphs are presented here, along with some preliminary analysis.

While most BOB members were "graduates" of Loma Linda, we had, at that time, hundreds of members who were treated at

UFHPTI, MGH, MD Anderson and MPRI. They are represented in the survey results.

Urinary function: Eighty percent, or 1,156 members, said they didn't see any change in urinary function. Eighteen percent (259) said they did experience a change. Once again, here's one place where I could have asked a better question.

Members reported both positive and negative changes. Some reported temporary increases in urinary urgency or burning during urination after treatment ended. Just about all the urinary "problems" reported were temporary in nature.

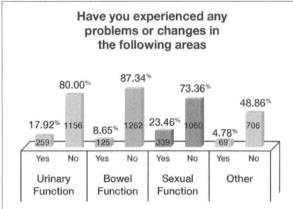

On the plus side, most of the respondents who answered "Yes" to this question indicated the change was positive: They no longer had to get up at night, or they got up less frequently, or their stream had improved. Some indicated that they no longer needed to take Flomax or other drugs for urinary function, medications they had been taking prior to treatment.

Two respondents who had surgery prior to proton therapy and another who had cryotherapy following a cancer recurrence reported incontinence. Others reported temporary urgency that disappeared over time. Very few experienced urinary urgency a year or two after treatment ended.

Bowel Function: Almost 9 percent indicted some change in bowel function after treatment. Most in this category reported some temporary rectal bleeding that resolved itself over time. A few reported temporary bowel urgency or more frequent bowel movements for some months after treatment.

One individual who had cryotherapy for a cancer recurrence after proton therapy reported serious, Grade 4 gastrointestinal complications.

Sexual Function: Seventy-three percent reported no change in sexual function. Twenty-three percent indicated changes had occurred. These changes ranged from slight to significant, including impotence. Many in the latter category were on hormonal therapy. Two noted that their impotence was caused by surgery prior to proton therapy.

Many of the 23 percent reported that erections were more difficult or were not as firm as before treatment.

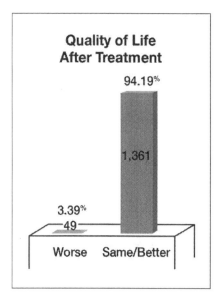

A few reported that ejaculation was painful for a few weeks to a few months after treatment. And some reported less ejaculate or no ejaculate.

Paraphrasing what several members said, "Erections aren't as firm as before treatment, but I'm also a few years older . . . in my 70s, or 80s."

Quality of Life After Treatment: As you can see from the bar chart, 94 percent reported that, following proton therapy, the quality of their lives was the same as, or better than before treatment. Just over 3 percent said the quality of their lives was worse.

The following comment by one member sums it up for many of those who responded:

"I never felt any side effects during or after treatment. I now can urinate like a teenager and my sex life is great."

Treatment Decision: As the chart indicates, almost 99 percent of those who chose proton therapy felt they made the right treatment decision. Fewer than 1 per-cent felt they did not. Similarly, 97 percent said they would make the same decision again, while fewer than 1 percent said they would not.

To put this in perspective, an August 2008 *New York Times* article reported that a survey showed that 20 percent of men who had chosen robotic surgery regretted their decision.

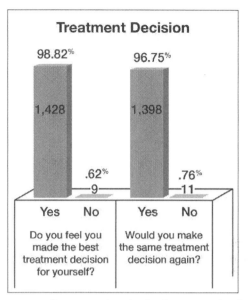

Rating Treatment Experience: About 96 percent rated their treatment experience in the outstanding range, while 0.35 percent said their treatment experience was poor.

Overall, how would you rate your treatment experience?

	Overall, how would you rate your treatment experience?							
	Outst.				Medium			Poor
%	90.10%	6.02%	2.28%	0.42%				0.35%
#	1,302	87	2	6				5

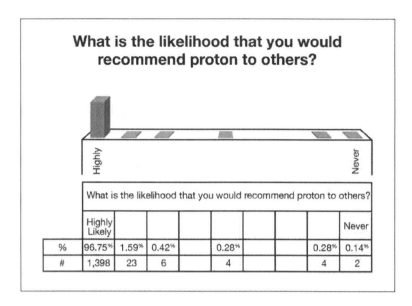

What is the likelihood that you would recommend proton to others?

	What is the likelihood that you would recommend proton to others?							
	Highly Likely							Never
%	96.75%	1.59%	0.42%		0.28%		0.28%	0.14%
#	1,398	23	6		4		4	2

Recommending Proton to Others: Once again, the overwhelming majority (98 percent) said it was highly likely they would recommend proton therapy to others. Fewer than 0.5 percent said they wouldn't. And 97 percent indicated they had already recommended proton therapy to relatives, friends or acquaintances.

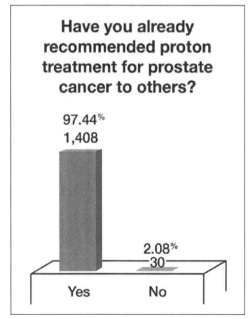

Have you already recommended proton treatment for prostate cancer to others?

97.44%
1,408

2.08%
30

Yes   No

But – Did It Work? After the results started coming in, I realized I forgot to ask an important question about whether or not their cancer was in remission. And the fact that I forgot to ask that question says a lot. Most of us truly believe that our cancer has been cured and we've gotten on with our lives. But the question must be asked.

I struggled with the wording, because cancer is an insidious disease. How do we know we're cured? Cancer of any kind may recur years after treatment. And with any treatment, those who are only a few months or even a couple of years post-treatment are never sure. So, in my second (one-question) survey, I asked, *"As far as you know*, has your proton treatment eliminated your prostate cancer?"

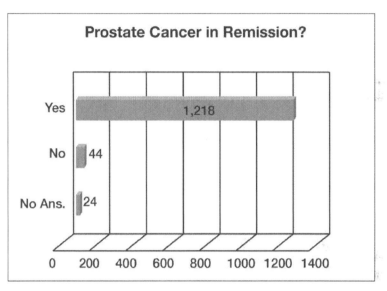

Prostate Cancer in Remission?

Although we didn't provide a comment section for this question, I received dozens of emails from members with lots of interesting commentary. Paraphrasing the most common response, it was, "Yes, I'm cured. Thank God for proton therapy." But there were many other comments.

One individual said, "I chose not to answer that question because it has only been two years since my treatment. My PSA is dropping nicely, but I won't know for sure until many years after treatment."

Another said, "It's been a year since my treatment ended. My PSA is dropping fast, so I answered, 'Yes'"

And another said, "My PSA is falling, but hasn't yet reached its nadir, so I answered, 'No.'"

Even with this variability in respondents' perspectives, the results are as follows: Out of 1,286 responses, 1,218, or 95 percent indicated they felt proton therapy had destroyed their prostate cancer; 44, or 3.4 percent indicated either it didn't eliminate their cancer, they had a recurrence, or they really didn't know yet, and 24 (1.8 percent) didn't provide an answer. Keep in mind, our membership consisted of men who were treated from just a few months to 19 years before we conducted the survey.

Summary: This was by no means a scientific survey. It had many flaws. But it did sample a remarkably large percentage of the prostate cancer proton population, and you can't deny the fact that proton therapy eliminates prostate cancer *at least* as well as any of the alternatives, and for the overwhelming majority of us who were fortunate enough to have had this treatment, our quality of life has been preserved.

I am in regular contact with men who have chosen alternative treatment modalities. And while most have had excellent results with disease-free survival, the quality-of-life stories I hear from so many of them are far different from what this survey tells us about proton therapy.

Perhaps the greatest testament to the superiority of proton therapy is that former patients band together to promote this treatment to family, friends, acquaintances and anyone else who will listen. You will not find this with surgery, seeds or IMRT.

2014 NAPT Survey

In 2014, the National Association for Proton Therapy commissioned Dobson DaVanzo & Associates, a healthcare consulting firm, to investigate clinical results and patient satisfaction among men treated with proton therapy for prostate cancer. They were asked to compare these results to those from a 2013 survey.

Survey Design

This survey was carefully designed by a team of clinicians and experts in the field. It incorporates questions from several validated survey instruments designed to capture information related to patients' satisfaction with their cancer treatment including the Assessment of Patient Experience of Cancer Care (APECC) developed by the National Cancer Institute, and the Consumer Assessment of Healthcare Providers and Systems (CAHPS) Cancer Care Survey developed by the Agency for Healthcare Research and Quality (AHRQ). The Expanded Prostate Cancer Index Composite (EPIC) was also used to measure each patient's post-treatment health status. The survey was field tested with a group of proton therapy patients, including several BOB members, who provided valuable feedback that was incorporated into the final survey instrument.

The survey was designed to capture important information about disease-free survival as well as specific quality-of-life results. Information was collected on patient demographics, pretreatment conditions, why patients chose proton therapy, patient satisfaction, and much more.

Large Response – Excellent Patient Population Representation

In total, about 3,800 former patients from 12 proton centers responded to the survey. To put this in perspective, this was twice the number that responded to the previous survey, with five additional proton centers represented. It represents approximately 17 percent of all patients who received proton therapy for prostate cancer since this treatment modality had been introduced. Many who responded to this survey were treated 10, 15, and even 20 (or more) years prior to the survey. So, this was certainly an excellent representation of the prostate cancer proton population at that time.

Almost 70 percent of respondents were college graduates. This is more than quadruple the national average for men in this age group, indicating that highly educated men seem to research their treatment options more thoroughly and they tend to gravitate to proton therapy.

Key Findings

As in the previous survey, patients reported great satisfaction with their proton therapy treatment:

- 98 percent believed they made the best treatment decision for themselves.
- 96 percent had recommended proton therapy to others.
- 98 percent rated their proton therapy as "excellent" (88 percent) or "good" (10 percent).
- 96 percent were "satisfied" (15 percent) or "extremely satisfied" (81 percent) with their proton therapy treatment.
- 85 percent reported their quality of life was "better than" (27 percent) or "the same as" (58 percent) before their treatment.
- Those patients who received proton only (i.e. no additional photon or hormonal therapy) reported urinary, bowel, and sexual function outcomes consistent with a cancer-free control group that *never* had any treatment for prostate cancer. This is significant.

Perhaps most significant is the following:

- Overall, 97 percent reported no recurrence of their prostate cancer – slightly higher for those recently treated, and slightly lower for those treated 10 or more years ago.

According to the Dobson DaVanzo report, this compares quite favorably with a study of long-term outcomes with IMRT, where a study published in the *Journal of Urology* [176 (4):1415-1419] reported an 11 percent recurrence rate eight years after treatment.

As expected, those who received treatment beyond proton therapy, such as photon treatment or hormonal therapy had lower bowel, sexual, and hormonal health related quality of life (HRQOL) scores compared to those receiving only proton therapy, once again, supporting the fact that proton therapy does an outstanding job targeting the tumor volume and minimizing radiation to surrounding healthy tissue. This is also one more case for catching the disease early, because as prostate cancer progresses, more aggressive treatments are required to control the disease.

Why Did Respondents Choose Proton Therapy?

According to the survey, the most common reasons for choosing proton therapy over surgery, conventional radiation (IMRT), or brachytherapy (seeds) were fewer expected bowel side effects, sexual side effects, and urinary side effects.

Final Comment on the NAPT Survey

In the past I had been critical of retrospective studies that used Medicare billing records over a two-year period to draw conclusions on patient outcomes. These studies typically concluded that proton therapy was no better than IMRT. The above survey represents a large population of patients, treated at multiple proton centers, over a 24-year period. It's all *patient-reported* data, and it confirms what the science suggests, namely, if you increase the dose of radiation to the tumor and reduce the dose to healthy tissue, you can expect higher cure rates and fewer side effects.

Provision/Bryant Survey Compares Proton Therapy to Seeds, Conventional Radiation and Surgery

Provision Healthcare commissioned Bryant Research to conduct a survey comparing patient satisfaction levels with selected prostate cancer treatment modalities. The survey was developed in conjunction with Provision leadership using a nationally listed sample of patients. It focused on patients between ages 50 and 75 with a history of prostate cancer who were at least 12 months post-treatment. They collected data on patient-reported quality-of-life measures after treatment.

The sample targets were 200 patients each, who had chosen surgery, conventional (X-ray) radiation, brachytherapy (seeds) and proton therapy. The survey was conducted between 2013 and 2015. Here are some of the findings from the survey reported in 2016:

- While most participants felt a second opinion on treatment options was important, the proton therapy group was significantly more likely to characterize a second opinion as "very important" than all others.

- Roughly half those who chose a treatment modality *other* than proton therapy indicated they were unfamiliar with proton therapy.
- Most of the respondents in each treatment group indicated they held a positive impression of their chosen treatment modality.
- Those who chose proton therapy were more positive (97 percent positive) about their choice than those who elected another course of treatment.
- Except for those who elected radical prostatectomy, respondents were more negative about surgery than any of the other options listed, with the proton therapy patient group expressing the most negativity toward surgery.
- Proton therapy patients placed *significantly* higher importance than those in all the other groups on each of the following aspects:
  - Overall quality of life
  - Ability to control urinary function after treatment
  - Living life the way I want after treatment
- Proton patients also rated the importance of maintaining sexual function significantly higher than those who chose conventional radiation.
- Proton therapy patients (97 percent) were significantly more likely to recommend their treatment option to other men with a prostate cancer diagnosis than those who experienced the other types of treatment were to recommend their choice:
  - Brachytherapy (70 percent)
  - Conventional radiation (67 percent)
  - Surgery (57 percent)
- Proton therapy patients (97 percent) also were significantly more likely to say they would select the same treatment option should they have to make the decision today, than those who experienced other treatment options:
  - Brachytherapy (68 percent)
  - Radiation (66 percent)
  - Surgery (26 percent)

- Overall, proton therapy patients reported the best outcomes with respect to maintaining sexual function after treatment.
- Proton therapy patients were significantly more likely than radiation or surgery patients to report treatment did not interfere with their overall quality of life after treatment.
- Proton therapy patients were significantly more likely than all others to report treatment did not interfere with the ability to control urinary function after treatment.

Much Lower Probability of Secondary Cancers

Because proton therapy is so precise in delivering cancer killing radiation to the target (tumor), very little radiation is delivered to normal, healthy tissue. The *Prostate Cancer Communication Newsletter* (Volume 23, Number 1, March 2007) reported that with proton therapy, healthy tissue sees 3 -5 times *less* radiation than with IMRT. The authors conclude:

"The physical characteristics of protons guarantee that for any given treatment plan they will always result in a lower total radiation dose to normal tissue than can be achieved with any form of X-ray therapy, which over a century's worth of clinical experience in radiation oncology has been shown to always be beneficial to the patient."

Dr. Andrew Lee, while at the MD Anderson Cancer Center in Houston, TX said, "We found that proton therapy may decrease the rates of second radiogenic cancers by up to 30-40 percent compared to IMRT" (Fontenot et al. IFROBP 2009). This is corroborated by the clinical experience at Massachusetts General Hospital: When they reviewed their secondary cancer rates with protons, the rates were significantly lower than the national average with X-rays, and interestingly, the patients who received proton therapy alone (not mixed X-rays and protons) had zero second malignancies (C. Chung ASTRO 2007).

Another Opinion on Secondary Cancers

The International Journal of Cancer (2008; 123:1141-45) reported that the risk of developing secondary colon cancers is 3.4 times greater with men who have received radiation treatment for prostate cancer. The interesting point here is that this could not have included men who were treated with proton therapy, as the colon sees virtually zero radiation with proton therapy, whereas the colon is routinely exposed to photon radiation during other radiotherapy modalities, including IMRT.

According to the study, there is no increase in the incidence of rectal cancer with men undergoing radiation therapy for prostate cancer.

Proton Therapy vs. Surgery

As reported in the *University of Florida Precision Newsletter*, March 19, 2014, physicians and researchers followed hundreds of prostate cancer patients treated with protons for early-, intermediate- and advanced-prostate cancer. At five years, 99 percent of men with early and intermediate disease are cancer free, and 76 percent of men with advanced disease were cancer free[1]. Following is a table reprinted with permission of UF Health Proton Therapy Institute (UFHPTI) comparing five-year proton results with published surgery results. The numbers speak for themselves.

Decision Points	Proton Therapy for Prostate Cancer	Surgery for Prostate Cancer
Disease Control[*]	99%-76%[1]	84%-60%[2,3]
Treatment		
Major complication rate	1%[1**]	28.6%[4]
Invasive Procedure	No	Yes
Long Recovery Time	No	Yes
Fatigue	No	Yes
30-day mortality rate	0%	0.5%[4]
Rehospitalization rate	0% (N/A)	4.5%[4]
Side Effects Percent of patients who experience a change post treatment		
Incontinence	0%[1]	6%-30%[4]
Impotence	34%[1]	60%-80%[1]
Inguinal hernia	0% (N/A)	7%-21%[4]
Fecal Incontinence	1.4%[1]	17%-32%[5]

*Disease control is defined as freedom from clinical or PSA progression at five years.
**1% per Common Terminology Criteria for Adverse Events (CTCAE) v4.0; 5.3% per CTCAE v3.0

1.Mendenhall, NP et al. Five-Year Outcomes from 3 Prospective Trials of Image-Guided Proton Therapy for Prostate Cancer. Int J Radiation Oncol Biol Phys 2014 March; 88(3):596-602.

2.Han, M et al. Long-Term Biochemical Disease-Free and Cancer-Specific Survival Following Anatomic Radical Retropubic Prostatectomy: The 15-Year Johns Hopkins Experience. Urol Clin North Am 2001 Aug; 28(3):555-65.

3.Qi, P et al. Long-Term Oncological Outcomes of Men Undergoing Radical Prostatectomy With Preoperative Prostate-Specific Antigen <2.5 ng/mL and 2.5-4 ng/mL. Urol Oncol 2013 Nov; 31(8):1527-32.

4.Treatment Option Overview for Prostate Cancer, Health Professional Version, http://www.cancer.gov/cancertopics/pdq/treatment/prostate/ HealthProfessional/page3#Section_2223. Retrieved Aug. 28, 2013.

5.Bishoff JT et al. Incidence of fecal and urinary incontinence following radical perineal and retropubic prostatectomy in a national population. J Urol 160 (2): 454-8, 1998.

Proton Therapy vs. IMRT

The following tables are also presented with permission from UFHPTI. Once again, the tables speak for themselves. Most noteworthy is the fact that disease control numbers are markedly higher with proton therapy.

Standard Fractionation Protocol

A comparison of published data on patients treated with protons at UFHPTI compared with IMRT patients treated at Memorial Sloan Kettering (MSK) and Mayo Clinic (Mayo) showed quite favorable disease-free survival results with protons for low-, intermediate- and high-risk patients. Reported data was for five or more years since treatment. Gastrointestinal (GI) and Genitourinary (GU) morbidity (side effects) were comparable. Not shown in the table are bowel urgency results, where proton showed a remarkable advantage at 7 percent vs. IMRT at 15 percent.

Prostate Cancer ≥5Y reported outcomes of contemporary standard fractionation IMRT & Proton Therapy (UFHealth)				
Biochem. Freedom from Progression	MSK[1] IMRT (1002)	Mayo[4] IMRT (302)	UF[2] **Proton** (211)	UF[3] **Proton** (1327)
Dose/#	86Gy/48f	73.8/41f	78CGE/39	78CGE/39
Low Risk	98%	77%	**99%**	**99%**
Int. Risk	86%	70%	**99%**	**94%**
High Risk	68%	53%	**76%**	**74%**
Gr 3+ GI	0.7%	0[4]	0.5%	0.6%
Gr 3+ GU	2.2%	0.7%	1.0%	2.9%

[1]Spratt et al, 2013 IJROBP. Long-term outcomes . . . . IMRT. 81Gy/45 fx
[2]Mendenhall et al, 2014, IJROBP. Five Year Outcomes, 3 prospective trials
[3]Bryant et al, IJROBP 95: 2016. Five Year Outcomes >1300 men, 78CGE/39 fx
[4]Vora et al, ... 75.6 Gy/42 fx, toxicity at last FU

Hypofractionation Studies

In comparing hypofractionation patients (higher doses, fewer treatments), as the table below shows, disease-free survival at five or more years for low- to high-risk patients is better with proton therapy than with IMRT at Radiation Therapy Oncology Group (RTOG). Also, GI and GU morbidity is markedly lower with proton therapy. These results are significant.

Prostate Cancer: ≥5Y reported outcomes of moderate hypofractionation IMRT & proton therapy: 70Gy/CGE in 28 fx (UFHealth)		
Biochem. Freedom from Progression	RTOG[1] IMRT N=550	UF[2] Proton N=228
Low risk	86.3%	**99%**
Int risk	--	**93%**
Gr 3+ GI[3]	4.1%	0.5%
Gr 3+ GU[3]	3.5%	1.7%
[1]Lee et al, 2016, J Clin Oncol, Randomized ... Two Fractionation .. Low Risk ... 79% got IMRT and 21% got CRT evenly balanced between fractionation arms [2]Henderson et al, 2017, ACTCA Oncologica. [3]At med 5.8y, late Gr3+GI and GU complications were higher in the hypofractionation arm HR 1.31-1.59 than in the conventional arm, which delivered 73.8 Gy in 41 fractions		

More Reasons to Avoid Surgery

Conversation with Prominent Oncologist

In a conversation with a prominent oncologist who specializes in treating prostate cancer, he told me, "With surgery you can never be sure you removed all the prostate tissue. The prostate gland is not that well defined. So, there could be – and often is – untreated, cancerous prostate tissue left behind. The seminal vesicles, for example are very small and hard to see, like cellophane." He further stated, "With nerve-sparing surgery, doctors are intentionally leaving behind tissue that can be cancerous. Maybe that's one reason why there are 35 percent failures with surgery in 10 years." A big advantage with protons is that they treat the prostate, the capsule, the seminal vesicles plus a margin around that entire target volume.

Avoiding Surgical Mistakes

ProPublica published an article in September 2013, titled, *How Many Die from Medical Mistakes in U.S. Hospitals?* It could be at least 210,000 patients a year, according to the study. In 2010, the Office of Inspector General for Health and Human Services said that hospital care errors contributed to the deaths of 180,000 patients in Medicare alone in one year.

The Journal of Patient Safety in 2013, stated the numbers may be much higher − "between 210,000 and 440,000 patients each year who go to the hospital for care suffer some type of preventable harm that contributes to their death," according to their study.

No one knows for sure what the exact number is, but clearly, it's a substantial number of patients who are harmed. A significant percentage of these are surgery patients. About 1,300 times a year, surgeons operate on the wrong person or remove the wrong limb or organ. Also, surgical instruments are left inside patients about once in every 5,000 surgeries.

Parade Magazine reported that far more common are stitches coming loose, blood clots forming and infections happening. The Centers for Disease Control and Prevention reports that 99,000 patients a year die from hospital-borne infections and that more than a quarter of a million pressure ulcers (bed sores) are reported each year.

Tip: There are many times when surgery is the only option or is the best option for treating a medical condition. But always consider the non-invasive option if your research convinces you the results will be comparable.

"Is Proton Therapy a Breakthrough for Cancer Patients?"

This is the title of an article published on May 30, 2109, in GlobalVillageSpace.com. According to researchers, new studies show that while cure rates for X-ray therapy and proton therapy are similar, the risk of severe side effects is much lower with proton therapy.

Dr. Brian C. Baumann, a radiation oncologist at the Washington University School of Medicine, in St. Louis, MO, is the lead author of the study. He and his team presented their findings at the American Society of Clinical Oncology's (ASCO) annual meeting in Chicago, IL in June 2019.

Researchers in this study looked at 1,500 cancer patients who were receiving a combination of chemotherapy and radiation therapy for localized cancers of several types, including lung, brain, head, neck, gastrointestinal and gynecological cancers. The study found that the risk of severe side effects within 90 days of treatment was two-thirds lower for people who received proton therapy, compared with those who received X-ray radiation.

The article concluded with, "One might suggest that this therapy is a Godsend for cancer patients braving through their painful and draining radiation therapy."

Summary

Once again, all doctors and scientists agree. The only safe dose of radiation to heathy tissue is a zero dose. And, of all the radio-therapy options available for treating cancer, proton beam therapy comes the closest to that goal.

The growing body of evidence continues to show what the laws of physics predict, namely, that proton therapy destroys cancer as well as all X-ray models, and does so with minimal radiation deposited on healthy tissue, thus minimizing the likelihood of side effects or secondary cancers later in life.

CHAPTER 16

Latest Developments in Proton Therapy

"Don't worry about getting perfect, just keep getting better."

– Frank Peretti

34 Proton Centers in the U.S.

A lot has changed since the first edition of my book was published. When I was treated in late 2000 there was only one proton center in the U.S., Loma Linda University Cancer Center in Southern California. As of this writing, almost 20 years later, there are 34 proton centers in the U.S. with at least nine more in development. See Appendix for a complete list of proton centers in the U.S.

The following graphic shows the location of these centers.

Proton Centers in the U.S.

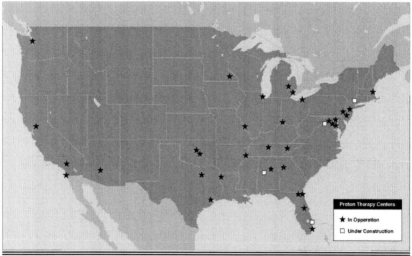

Image by Mark Hickey, Marcus Design Group

34 Proton Centers in the U.S. 84 Centers Worldwide

Today, most prospective proton patients in the U.S. live within a day's drive of a proton therapy center. Even so, fewer than 2 percent of men being treated for prostate cancer are receiving this extraordinary treatment, and fewer than 0.5 percent for all other cancers. The obstacles that patients face today in accessing proton therapy have changed, but are still significant.

In addition to the 34 operating proton centers in the U.S. there are an additional 50 proton centers in 18 other countries, for a total of 84 proton centers worldwide, with 39 under construction and 21 in planning stages. For a complete listing of proton centers worldwide, visit the Particle Therapy Co-Operative Group (PTCOG) website, https://www.ptcog.ch.

More than 140 Disease Sites Being Treated with Proton Therapy

While prostate cancer, breast cancer, lung cancer and brain cancers are most commonly treated, many other cancers and conditions are routinely treated with proton therapy. More than 140 disease sites are treated, including acoustic neuromas, meningiomas,

220

chordomas and chondrosarcomas, arteriovenous malformations (AVMs), pituitary adenomas, uveal melanomas (eye), nasopharynx and oropharynx (head and neck), pancreatic carcinomas and many more. Just about any solid tumor can be treated with proton therapy.

Proton therapy has turned out to be an ideal way of treating tumors in children. Because of the proton beam's incredible accuracy and ability to destroy tumors without doing collateral damage, it's been proven to be especially effective in treating pediatric cancers.

Conventional (X-ray) radiation has always been effective in treating pediatric cancers. But the collateral damage to surrounding healthy organs and tissue can have a devastating impact on a child, including stunted growth of limbs, and secondary cancers later in life.

Pencil Beam Technology

As precise as the original passive-beam technology is, newly developed pencil beam, or active beam scanning (ABS) technology is even more precise. The pencil beam uses an electronically guided scanning system and magnets to deliver a pinpoint beam that can be precisely delivered to the target in three dimensions.

Pencil beam technology allows doctors to treat large tumors that were previously out-of-field range of passive beam systems. It also lends itself nicely to treating amorphous, non-symmetrical tumors.

Some of the newer proton centers have both passive beam and pencil beam treatment rooms. A few have pencil beam only.

Whether pencil beam is superior to passive beam for treating prostate cancer is a matter of opinion. There are radiation oncologists on both sides of this issue. Some believe that, since the pencil beam is more precise, it should do a better job treating prostates. Others believe that since the prostate is essentially a symmetrical target, the passive beam is superior because the passive beam penumbra does a better job treating the edges of the target volume. Bottom line: prostate cancer patients are well served with both treatment forms.

Both forms of proton therapy, in my opinion, are superior to IMRT or any other form of conventional X-ray radiotherapy precisely because of the Bragg peak and the markedly lower dose of radiation deposited on healthy tissue around the target.

Robotic Patient Positioning

Proper patient positioning is key to properly focusing the beam on the tumor each day. Until recently, patient positioning was a process involving several steps and multiple radiation technicians. The use of robotics significantly shortens patient prep time, improves accuracy of the delivered beam, and increases productivity (can treat more patients).

Single Treatment Room Proton Centers

One of the largest barriers to entry into proton treatment has been the excessively high capital cost of building large, multi-treatment room proton centers, each with three-story gantries surrounded by thick concrete and steel walls, along with complex control systems. Costs for these centers sometimes exceeded $200 million. Early proton centers were said to be, "as large as a football field." While this is an exaggeration, it isn't far off the mark.

Several companies have successfully designed and developed single-room treatment centers for a fraction of the cost of multi-room centers. And, while multi-room treatment centers are still being built, most new centers are single-room design, allowing more affordable proton centers to be built in locations all over the world.

Hypofractionation Clinical Trials

Hypofractionation (HF) was discussed in an earlier chapter. This fast-emerging technology is showing great promise. Almost all proton centers are either involved in clinical trials using HF or are offering HF as a treatment option to patients with early stage cancer. This technology is expected to improve dramatically in the coming years, with higher and higher safe doses of proton particles delivered over fewer treatment fractions.

Capacity for Fewer than 1 Percent of Radiation Patients

Despite the explosive growth of proton therapy and the large and growing number of proton centers being built, there still isn't enough worldwide proton capacity to treat all the patients who could benefit from this technology.

It's estimated that about half the number of patients who receive radiation treatment would be better served – i.e. improved disease-free survival and quality of life after treatment – by having proton therapy. Yet, capacity exists for treating fewer than 1 percent of those patients.

This is expected to change in the coming years for the following reasons:

1. Cost to build proton treatment centers is coming down.

2. Hypofractionation (higher dose – fewer treatments) is expected to reduce treatment costs and treatment time considerably.

3. Ongoing clinical trials are expected to show clearly the benefits of proton therapy over conventional radiation, resulting in better insurance coverage, higher patient demand and more proton centers being built.

National Association for Proton Therapy (NAPT) and Lifetime Achievement Award

NAPT, an independent, nonprofit organization, was founded in 1990. Initially its purpose was to educate and increase awareness about the clinical benefits of proton therapy; to ensure patient access to this important treatment modality; and to encourage cooperative research and innovation to advance cost-effective utilization of proton therapy.

Over the years it has grown to become the strongest voice for proton therapy, perhaps in the world with membership representing virtually all proton centers in the U.S. Thousands of cancer patients have benefited from the extraordinary work and active participation by the dedicated members of NAPT.

For the past several years, Deb and I have participated, as members, in NAPT activities, including attendance at the annual National Proton Conferences where both of us have been speakers.

In 2016, I was surprised and greatly honored to have been selected by NAPT to receive a Lifetime Achievement Award for:

"Pioneering and voluntary leadership in improving the lives of thousands of prostate cancer patients, through founding and leadership of The Brotherhood of the Balloon, the largest prostate cancer patient-advocacy organization in the world, and for writing the seminal book for educating the public on prostate cancer awareness, prevention, treatment and proton therapy."

I'm proud to be one of six people to have received this prestigious award, including NAPT founder and first executive director, Len Arzt, and proton pioneers, Dr. James Slater, Loma Linda University Cancer Center, Dr. James Cox, professor emeritus at MD Anderson Cancer Center, Dr. Herman Suit, founding Chairman of Radiation Oncology at Massachusetts General Hospital and Dr. George Laramore, professor, Radiation Oncology Department at Seattle Cancer Care Alliance.

CHAPTER 17

Diagnostic Tools, Techniques and Recent Developments

"Diagnosis is not the end, but the beginning of practice."

– Martin H. Fischer

The Big PSA Controversy

Before delving into the new and exciting developments in diagnostics, it's important that we talk about PSA screening. Opinions on this subject vary immensely. No wonder men are confused about prostate cancer detection. It's hard to find two doctors who agree on the value and importance of PSA testing for prostate cancer screening.

Just look at the differences of opinion between the "authorities" on prostate cancer screening:

American Cancer Society: Average-risk men with at least a 10-year life expectancy should begin discussions about prostate cancer screening at age 50 (younger for higher-risk men). Men with PSA less than 2.5 ng/mL may be retested every two years. Men with PSA greater than 2.5 ng/mL should be screened annually

American College of Physicians: Men ages 50 – 69 should discuss the risks and benefits of screening with their doctor. Average-risk men younger than age 50 and older than age 69, or any man with a life expectancy less than 10 – 15 years, should not be screened.

American Urological Association: Men ages 55 – 69 should discuss the risks and benefits of screening with their physician. Screening is not recommended for men younger than age 55, older than age 70, or anyone with a life expectancy of less than 10 – 15 years. Screening may be done every two years or less frequently, rather than annually.

National Comprehensive Cancer Network: Men with at least a 10-year life expectancy should begin discussions about screening at age 45. Screening remains an option for very healthy men over age 70. Men ages 45 – 49 with PSA greater than 1.0 ng/mL and men age 50 and older with PSA less than 3.0 ng/mL and no other indications for biopsy should repeat testing every one to two years. Men ages 40 – 49 with PSA below 1.0 ng/mL should be rescreened at age 50.

U.S. Preventive Services Task Force: Regardless of age, men without prostate cancer symptoms should not be routinely screened for prostate cancer.

Does this clear things up for you? Of course not. And for those of us who have snaked our way through this maze to a diagnosis, it gets even more complicated. There are so many treatment options available and they're all so disparate: Cut it, cook it, freeze it, zap it, or – leave it alone.

How does one navigate through this convoluted mess? The answer to this question is one of the reasons I wrote this book.

Let's look at one more opinion on PSA screening: As mentioned earlier, in 2012, the U.S. Preventive Service Task Force (USPSTF) took their extreme position – recommending no screening whatsoever – as an over-reaction to the number of needless invasive biopsies and quality-of-life-changing aggressive treatments that were being performed on so many men with early stage, non-aggressive cancers.

But the problem wasn't over-testing, it was over-*treating*. Many doctors took the USPSTF's recommendations literally and stopped PSA screening their patients. The result was a significant increase in undetected aggressive prostate cancers over the past several years.

In the spring of 2017, the USPSTF softened their position somewhat on PSA testing and now recommends that, "the decision as to whether to undergo PSA-based screening should be made individually for each man aged 55 to 69 years, taking into account the man's values and clinical circumstances."

In 2018, Medscape reported that medical centers in the U.S. are seeing a decrease in low-grade prostate cancer and a significant increase in intermediate and high-risk disease. This correlates directly with the USPSTF recommendation to stop PSA screening in 2012.

My position on PSA screening

Although PSA isn't the perfect test, it's considered by most prominent urologic oncologists to be one of the most successful biomarkers in the history of oncology. Knowing that the PSA test is a non-specific test for detecting prostate cancer, it's still a valuable *relative* indicator and can be an early warning signal that you should pay attention to.

In my opinion, all men 50 and older should have annual PSA tests with no upper age limit (Note: One member of our group was diagnosed and treated at age 87. He lived 15 more years to 102). Men at higher risk (e.g. African American or close relative with prostate cancer) should begin PSA screening at age 40.

If PSA is high or is rising rapidly, a decision to proceed with a biopsy should be based on several factors, including PSA doubling time, age, life expectancy and the results of newer technology imaging, which will be discussed later in this chapter.

PSA Density as a Diagnostic Tool

PSA typically comes from two places: healthy prostate tissue and prostate cancer cells. Men with large prostates have more prostate tissue and typically produce more PSA regardless of whether prostate cancer is present. Some men with normal, or even low PSA levels, have been found to have prostate cancer. And some men with high PSA levels have been found to be cancer free.

Calculating PSA density can help doctors determine whether your PSA results are normal or possibly cancerous. PSA density is determined by dividing your PSA by your prostate size in milliliters (mL). A man with a PSA of 2.6 ng/mL, and a prostate volume of 35mL would have a PSA density of 2.6/35 = 0.074. A rule of thumb is that "normal" PSA density is about 0.15. Lower numbers are considered safer and higher numbers should be looked at more closely.

A man with a PSA of 8.7 and a prostate volume of 30 mL would have a PSA density of 0.29. And a man with a PSA of 11 and prostate volume of 80 mL would have a PSA density of 0.14. In these examples, the individual with the lower PSA has the more worrisome PSA density.

Some doctors believe that PSA density is a reasonably good tool to use for men with high PSAs, but not a very good predictor of cancer activity for men with PSAs below 4 ng/mL.

By using several tools, such as PSA density, PSA velocity and free-PSA, along with imaging tools to be discussed, doctors can better estimate your chances of having prostate cancer. The NCCN uses PSA density as one factor in their guidelines for choosing active surveillance vs. surgery or radiation for treating prostate cancer. Overall, men with high PSA density should be more vigilantly monitored for prostate cancer.

Note for clarification: prostate size can be expressed in milliliters (mL), cubic centimeters (cc) or grams. The first two measurements are volumetric measurements and they are equal, i.e. one milliliter equals one cubic centimeter. The third unit of measurement (grams) is a measure of weight. The human body is made up mostly of water, and since one gram of water is almost exactly one milliliter or one cubic centimeter in volume, you will find prostate size expressed in all three units: mL, cc and grams. For all practical purposes they are all equal: a 30 mL prostate = 30 cc = 30 grams.

Evolution of Prostate Cancer Testing, Detection

Until the mid-1980s – before the PSA test – the only way doctors could determine if a patient had prostate cancer, was to start with a digital rectal exam (DRE). If a lump or irregularity was felt, then a biopsy would be performed – without any imaging. Back then, this "totally blind biopsy" routinely missed cancer. Also, the transrectal needle biopsy often resulted in a high incidence of sepsis, bleeding, hospitalization, and infection.

An alternative was to do the biopsy through the perineum – the space between the rectum and testes. But to do this, the doctor would have to guide the needle with his finger inserted in the rectum to be sure it hit the prostate – a rudimentary and awkward procedure at best. And still, many cancers were missed.

Transrectal Ultrasound Guided Biopsy

The PSA test was a breakthrough when it received FDA approval in 1986. If rising PSA suggested the possibility of cancer, doctors would order a prostate biopsy.

An ultrasound machine was used to provide a cloudy image of the prostate while a hollow needle was passed through the rectal wall into the prostate to collect tissue samples. This was called transrectal ultrasound guided biopsy (TRUS). The transrectal ultrasound guided biopsy has been the standard prostate cancer detection procedure for more than 30 years.

The ultrasound imaging used for the biopsy allows doctors to visualize the prostate and any *significant* abnormalities, but it doesn't allow them to see small, potentially cancerous lesions that should be targeted with the needle. So, the test is largely a random sampling of the prostate, often called a "blind biopsy."

A typical biopsy today removes 12 samples – six from each lobe of the prostate. Since the needle samples less than one-half of 1 percent of the prostate, cancers often go undetected. And even when cancer is detected, doctors can't be sure they found the most aggressive cancer in the prostate.

So, if your biopsy results are negative, it doesn't necessarily mean there's no cancer present. And if your biopsy results are positive for cancer, it doesn't necessarily mean the doctor found the most aggressive cancer in your prostate. Earlier I mentioned that I had two biopsies that were negative before I was diagnosed by the third biopsy. The cancer was there all the time.

Renowned urologic oncologist, Dr. Raoul Concepcion, director of the Comprehensive Prostate Center in Nashville, TN, says, "Prostate ultrasound and biopsy are the weakest steps in the diagnosis (of prostate cancer)."

Multi-parametric MRI

Prostate MRIs have been performed for many years on prostate cancer patients. Early MRI technology provided clearer images of soft tissues in the body, including the prostate bed. This helped doctors determine if prostate cancer had spread outside the prostate and into the seminal vesicles or other nearby structures.

Most recently, higher resolution MRI technology has provided much more valuable information by helping to identify suspicious lesions within the prostate. In some cases, advanced MRI technology can be used to estimate the aggressiveness of the cancer and help determine if a biopsy is even necessary, saving money and eliminating the risks of the biopsy procedure.

Until recently, 1.5-Tesla multiparametric MRI was state-of-the art. Today even more advanced, 3-Tesla mp-MRI can be found in leading cancer centers. As one radiologist commented, "If a picture is worth a thousand words, a 3-T mp-MRI is an encyclopedia." The definition and clarity of the imaging allow doctors to see things never before visible with earlier imaging systems. This helps to ensure that the cancer will be found and that aggressive cancerous lesions won't be missed during biopsy.

The key is finding a medical center that has the latest, most advanced technology (3-T mp-MRI) and an experienced radiologist to interpret the test results, a challenge in today's world. Also, since the technology is still relatively new, not all private insurers cover the 3-T mp-MRI imaging test.

Bulletin: Coming in the not-too-distant future is 7-Tesla mp-MRI imaging.

PI-RADS

The term, PI-RADS, stands for Prostate Imaging Reporting and Data System. This is one more piece of data that comes from multiparametric MRI imaging. PI-RADS is an important classification system that uses a five-point scale to report on the likelihood of clinically significant prostate cancer. Most doctors consider prostate cancer to be clinically significant if the Gleason score is 7 or higher.

Following a multiparametric MRI, your doctor can give you your PI-RAD assessment, which would fall into one of the following categories:

PI-RADS 1   *Highly unlikely* that clinically significant cancer is present
PI-RADS 2   *Unlikely* that clinically significant cancer is present
PI-RADS 3   *Uncertain* whether clinically significant cancer is present
PI-RADS 4   *Likely* that clinically significant cancer is present
PI-RADS 5   *Highly likely* that clinically significant cancer is present

Typically, a biopsy would be recommended for results of PI-RADS 4 or 5. For results of PI-RADS 1 or 2, a recommendation for biopsy is considered inappropriate. For results of PI-RADS 3, a biopsy may be appropriate depending on factors such as patient history, patient and doctor preferences, and preferred standard of care.

Major Breakthrough: MRI Fusion-Guided and In-Bore Biopsies

A significant advancement made possible by mp-MRI is the MRI fusion-guided biopsy. This is a procedure where an mp-MRI image is overlaid (fused) onto an ultrasound image so the biopsy needle can be directed – via 3D high-definition image – to the suspicious areas identified by the MRI. This has shown to be extremely effective in targeting cancerous lesions in the prostate.

An even more advanced technology using mp-MRI involves doing real-time imaging *during* the biopsy, called in-bore MRI-guided biopsy. This, in my opinion is the current state-of-the-art in prostate imaging and prostate biopsy. The in-bore MRI-guided biopsy offers even more precision in finding and precisely sampling suspicious lesions during the biopsy. Both the MRI fusion-guided and in-bore MRI-guided biopsy procedures are costly and may not be covered by insurance.

Unfortunately, these technologies aren't in widespread practice as of this writing. The equipment required to image and register the MRI and ultrasound images is costly, and insurance reimbursement rates may not justify the investment for all hospitals. Also, not every community is blessed with radiologists who can interpret 3T mp-MRI images. Nevertheless, more and more medical institutions are purchasing the equipment, training staff, employing this technology, and are beginning to move up the steep learning curve.

In Europe, doctors are beginning to use advanced MRI imaging as a decision-making tool to determine whether or not to prescribe a biopsy. The U.S. is behind in this movement.

Good News, Bad News

The good news – as stated above – is that 3T mp-MRI, fusion-Guided and in-bore MRI-guided biopsy technology exists and is a *giant* improvement over the standard, "blind biopsy" procedure. The bad news is that accessibility to this exciting technology is limited. Most urologists are still using 30^+-year-old transrectal ultrasound-guided (blind) biopsies to look for prostate cancer.

Clearly, we're moving in the direction of using state-of-the-art imaging technology to find and stage cancers. No single test is perfect. But these advances are significant, and the latest technology provides much more information than ever before to help in diagnosing prostate cancer and in making critical treatment decisions.

In addition to 3-T mp-MRI technology and MRI-guided biopsies, newer, high-resolution ultrasound systems are also on the horizon. These should be of great benefit in targeting suspicious lesions during a needle biopsy. One significant benefit is that a radiologist is not required to read the high-resolution ultrasound images.

The time is coming when doctors will use these or similar technologies to determine if a patient with a rising PSA even needs an invasive biopsy.

I am convinced that the current state-of-the-art in prostate imaging is 3-tesla multi-parametric MRI (3T mp-MRI). And the corresponding state-of-the-art biopsy technique is 3T mp-MRI in-bore guided biopsy.

Tip: If I were a patient with rising PSA and my doctor felt a biopsy was necessary, then without hesitation I would find a way to have the real-time in-bore 3-T MRI procedure. This technique is infinitely more precise than the procedure that is routinely practiced, namely, transrectal ultrasound guided biopsy or TRUS (i.e. "blind biopsy"). A far better option than the TRUS is the MRI fusion-guided biopsy, but still not as good or as precise as the in-bore, real-time technique, in my opinion.

Meeting an MRI Guru

One of the premier practitioners of the 3T mp-MRI in-bore biopsy technique is Dr. Joseph Busch at the Busch Center in Alpharetta, GA. Dr. Busch was trained by the world's leading experts, Professors Jelle Barenstz, Jurgen Futterer and Anwar Padhani, in Europe; he's lectured and taught mp-MRI at RSNA, and Johns Hopkins; and is a member of ESUR, International Cancer Imaging Society and RSNA. Dr. Busch uses state-of-the-art, 4th generation 3T mp-MRI in his practice.

In late November 2019, Deb Hickey and I were invited to the grand opening of the new Busch Center, just outside of Atlanta, GA. We had the opportunity to spend some time with Dr. Busch and his wife, Kathy, who has been his partner in developing this technology for the past several years. Deb and I were astounded by their depth of knowledge and experience in this field. We left even more convinced that this procedure is the best available for detecting prostate cancer.

As mentioned earlier, this technology is available only at a few leading-edge medical centers in the world. In my opinion, it's worth the cost and inconvenience of traveling to a center that offers this technology for the benefits the patient receives, namely, precise real-time targeting of lesions/tumors within the prostate. The net result is the patient has a much better chance of his cancer being caught early. Additionally, there is a much better chance that the most aggressive cancer will be found with this imaging technique. This information allows doctors to custom design the right treatment protocol for the patient, giving him the best opportunity to have his cancer destroyed.

PET/CT Scans

These important imaging tests can be done on patients with suspected metastasis (cancer moved outside the prostate to another part of the body) or for patients with recurrent prostate cancer.

Four of these relatively new technologies include the Axumin PET/CT Scan, C-11 Choline PET/CT Scan, C-11 Acetate PET/CT Scan, and Gallium 68 PSMA PET/CT Scan.

CT stands for computerized tomography, commonly referred to as a CAT scan. CT scanners emit X-rays and generate cross-sectional images of anatomical structures. PET stands for positron emission tomography. PET scans measure metabolic activity and molecular function using a radioactive tracer. PET/CT is a hybrid imaging technique that's been proven to exhibit high diagnostic accuracy and is increasingly being used as a cancer staging tool.

Typically, a small amount of radioactive tracer is introduced into the body through an intravenous catheter (IV). A PET scanner detects the radioactive tracer's distribution and displays a computerized image on a computer monitor. These images are reviewed by radiologists to determine if cancer is present, to what degree, and exactly where it's located.

These state-of-the-art imaging technologies have the capability of finding metastatic or recurrent cancer at early stages and at low PSA levels, in some cases below 1.0 ng/mL. To my knowledge, all but the PSMA scan are FDA approved and reimbursable by medical insurers.

Avoiding Biopsies

Some medical centers use a combination of mp-MRI and PET/CT scan to gain a better perspective on the aggressiveness of suspected cancer activity to determine if a biopsy is even necessary. Important strides are being made with imaging technology and this will serve the patient well.

Bottom Line

If you have rising PSA that suggests the possibility of prostate cancer activity, it would be to your great advantage to find a medical center that can perform a 3-Tesla multi-parametric MRI of your prostate. This could tell you a) if a prostate biopsy is needed, and b) if so, exactly where the suspicious lesions are located so they can be targeted, sampled, and analyzed.

Under certain conditions as described above, PET/CT scans may also provide information that could be useful in diagnosing and staging your cancer.

By utilizing mp-MRI and PET/CT imaging you have a significantly greater chance of finding cancer if it's there, and ultimately selecting the best treatment for your condition.

CHAPTER 18

Ten Steps for Taking Control of The Detection and Treatment of Your Prostate Cancer

"Your life will fly by, so make sure you're the pilot."
— *Rob Liano*

Perhaps the most important message in this book is . . .

<u>You</u> are in charge of your health, and,
<u>You</u> should take control of your health.

This is *especially* important when dealing with prostate cancer. Starting with the diagnostic process all the way through to the treatment decision there is significant confusion, fueled by major differences of opinion among medical professionals and institutions. If you just do what your primary care physician or urologist suggests, you won't necessarily be making the best decision for *you*.

Take Control with These 10 Steps

If you follow these 10 steps, you'll greatly increase your chances of catching the disease early. The earlier prostate cancer is detected, the easier it is to cure.

Equally as important, once diagnosed, there are several things you can do that will virtually guarantee that you make the treatment decision that will give you the best chance of a cure as well as high quality of life after treatment. Here are the 10 steps:

237

1. Choose your doctors wisely.

2. Have a PSA test and DRE as part of your annual physical and track the results.

3. Have multi-parametric MRI imaging if PSA is rising.

4. Manage your biopsy test if above steps lead to a decision to schedule a biopsy.

5. Get a second opinion on your biopsy results.

6. Evaluate all treatment options – including active surveillance.

7. Talk with men (at least 10) who have been through each option you are considering.

8. Make your decision based on what is best for *you.*

9. Choose from among the best practitioners and treatment centers.

10. Maintain your physical and mental health.

1. Choose Your Doctors Wisely

Primary Care Physician: This is your first line of defense. Almost all prostate cancers are discovered as a result of action by the patient's family doctor. Too often cancer is discovered after it has progressed well beyond the early stage because the patient's doctor was not knowledgeable or didn't recognize the early signs of prostate cancer.

Many people choose a primary care doctor who's close to their home or office. Others move into a new neighborhood and make their choice based on a neighbor's recommendation. That may be a good start, but you should then meet with the doctor and conduct an interview to ensure that he or she is best for you.

My primary care physician's office is an hour and a half drive from my home. There are literally hundreds of doctors closer to where I live. I chose this physician for the following reasons:

- He's bright and personable.
- He spends time with his patients, carefully and thoughtfully answering all their questions. I'm never rushed through an annual physical or an office visit.
- He returns telephone calls within a reasonable time period.
- His specialty is gastroenterology, which is important to me, as both my parents and my sister had colon cancer, and this is another disease where heredity and early detection are critical factors.
- He has performed hundreds of colonoscopies, the most important early detection test for colon cancer.
- He understands the early signs of prostate cancer and is responsive to rising PSA.
- He keeps abreast of new developments in medicine.
- He is "proton friendly" and has recommended proton therapy to his patients.
- He came highly recommended by a doctor friend, whose opinion I value.

To me, it's worth the long drive to have the best medical care. If there were an emergency, I'd go to my local hospital emergency room. For everything else, I make the 1½-hour drive.

The principal function of your primary care physician should be *health protection* and *proactive disease prevention*. Good doctors won't wait for the telltale symptoms of a medical disorder to show up. They'll use all the information available to them – physical examinations, routine medical tests, and discussions with their patients – to probe for the earliest signs of a health problem.

Your automobile engine will run longer and smoother if you ensure the crankcase oil is clean and filled to the proper level and if you take other appropriate preventive maintenance measures. Waiting for the engine to "send you a signal" that something is wrong might be too late; the damage may already be done – and it may be irreversible.

Know your doctor's *opinion* of the PSA test. Many physicians believe that because PSA is a non-specific test for prostate cancer, a high or rising number isn't cause for alarm. Or they may feel PSA is of no concern until it progresses beyond the "normal" range. In both cases there may not be cause for *alarm*, but there *is* cause for *concern* and *action*. This is discussed in the next steps.

Most of us don't see a urologist until a problem is detected or suspected. So, your family doctor or primary care physician is your first line of defense against prostate cancer. Choose him or her wisely.

Proof of His/Her Competency: One side-story on my primary care doctor: My son-in-law was experiencing stomach pain over a two-week period. He visited his own doctor several times during that time and was told it was probably a stomach bug. When it persisted, his doctor prescribed an antibiotic.

For days thereafter, as my son-in-law was still in pain, I suggested he meet with my primary care physician. Within three days, my doctor diagnosed him with advanced, metastatic, neuroendocrine carcinoma of the pancreas – yes, advanced, metastatic pancreatic cancer, a devastating diagnosis with a terrible prognosis. Our lives were turned upside down.

What happened next was nothing short of a miracle. Through chemotherapy, diet changes, extraordinary care by my daughter, Deb, *and tons of prayers*, my son-in-law survived. Today, almost six years later, there's no evidence of cancer. Had my son-in-law gone another week undiagnosed, he likely would have died. My primary care doctor not only diagnosed the illness quickly, he also recommended the specialist oncologist who directed his vigorous treatment program. That's what a premier primary care physician can do.

Urologist: Sooner or later just about everyone, male or female, will need a urologist. Why wait until a problem develops? Why not do some homework and select your urologist before there's a medical need? He/she might not be taking new patients when you need him/her the most. The best time to select a good urologist is when you don't need one.

"The best time to select a good urologist is when you don't need one."

240

Most general practitioners are affiliated with a specific urologist and will typically refer their patients to this associate. That urologist may or may not be the best one for you.

If you have prostate cancer in your family, or if you have rising PSA, you should begin the search for a urologist at the earliest opportunity. Find out what doctors your friends and acquaintances use. Check their credentials. What hospital are they affiliated with? What is the reputation of that hospital? What technique do they use to take biopsy samples? How many biopsy core samples do they take? It should be a minimum of 12, preferably 20. Is a local anesthetic used during biopsy sampling?

Speak with patients who use the urologist you're considering. Especially speak with patients who've had prostate biopsies done by this doctor.

Find out if the doctor uses an assistant while taking biopsy samples. This is essential if you want the procedure to be done quickly, efficiently, and with the least amount of discomfort.

Find out if this doctor ever recommends anything other than surgery for prostate cancer patients who are younger than 65. Most urologists will suggest other treatment alternatives or active surveillance for older patients who can't tolerate the trauma of surgery, so the question is important: Does he/she ever recommend radiation, seeds, cryo, etc. to patients who are younger than 65?

You may not be able to find answers to all these questions but find out as much as you can.

One service *The Brotherhood of the Balloon* provides its members is a list of "proton-friendly" urologists within the U.S. These are doctors who have treated BOB members and are considered excellent physicians with open minds on proton therapy.

2. Have a PSA Test and DRE as Part of Your Annual Physical and Track the Results

This sounds pretty obvious, but it's surprising how many men are not paying attention to their PSA. Either they aren't having annual physicals, or they are having annual physicals, but their doctors have chosen not to run a simple PSA test or do a digital rectal exam (DRE). In other cases, the doctor is measuring PSA annually, but not communicating the results to the patient, or communicating to the patient, "Your PSA is within the 'normal' range." That's not enough. I receive calls all the time from men with advanced prostate cancer who fit into one of these categories.

Sad Example: A 54-year-old highly successful business owner called me with the following story. His last physical was several years ago. At that time, he had a PSA of 2.4 and a normal DRE. His next physical was six years later, at which time his PSA was 60, a DRE revealed a hard mass, and all 12 biopsy samples tested positive for adenocarcinoma, Gleason score 8. By not having routine physicals including monitoring PSA, this man put himself in an extremely vulnerable position with few options and a high risk of metastasis, for which there may be no cure.

A survey conducted by NOP Healthcare with 1,400 men in the U.S., U.K., France, Germany, Italy, Spain and Sweden showed one-third of men are not familiar with available tests to diagnose prostate cancer.

Second Sad Example: One of our members told me a story about his brother who had been having his PSA checked annually:

> *Ray made a life-changing mistake. He skipped his annual PSA test for reasons unknown to the family. Perhaps the federal government's guidelines deemphasizing PSA testing at the time had influenced his doctor's recommendation or my brother's thinking. He had no symptoms of prostate cancer.*
>
> *In early June 2016, he awakened one morning and couldn't urinate. He drove to the local hospital's emergency room. As part of the analysis they did blood work that revealed a PSA of 540. In two short years it had increased by a gigantic rate of 180 times!*

A biopsy showed aggressive prostate cancer. Multiple treatments were tried, including chemotherapy and androgen-deprivation therapy. None were able to arrest his prostate cancer. Less than six months later, Ray was dead.

Third Sad Example: Earlier in this book I wrote about a gentleman who was having annual physicals, which included a blood test including PSA measurement. And every year his doctor told him, "Everything is fine." One day, this same doctor told him he should see a urologist because his PSA had risen to 60!

242

This wasn't a single jump to 60, it had been rising steadily, but the doctor failed to recognize this and did nothing about it.

When this patient's urologist performed a biopsy, he found Gleason 10 advanced prostate cancer.

PSA May Help Predict Cancer

According to the Feb. 26, 2009 issue of *Johns Hopkins Health Alerts*, a study published in the *Journal of Oncology* (Vol. 25, p. 431) suggests that a man's PSA level measured when he is in his mid-40s to age 50 can predict whether he will develop prostate cancer up to 25 years later.

Researchers examined the records and blood samples of more than 21,000 men, age 50 and younger, and concluded that a man's total PSA level in middle age was the strongest predictor of developing prostate cancer. Younger men in this category with PSA level in the 0.5-1.0 range were 2.5 times more likely to develop prostate cancer. For those with PSA levels between 2 and 3 ng/mL (often considered to be within the "normal" range), the risk was more than 19 times higher.

Early Detection is the Key

The most important thing to remember about prostate cancer is that it is curable *if detected early*. Make sure you have a PSA test and DRE at least once a year. Competent primary care physicians will begin measuring their male patient's PSA around age 50 or 55, since prostate cancer is generally not found in men until after that age range. As mentioned in the previous chapter, my recommendation is to begin at age 50. And if there's prostate cancer in your family, begin measuring your PSA level at age 40 or sooner. It is wise to have an early "baseline" PSA, especially if you are at higher risk. The test is simple and inexpensive.

"Prostate cancer is curable if detected early."

If your PSA rises by more than 0.5 ng/mL in one year, consider repeating the test in three months to see if this trend is continuing or possibly accelerating. If the PSA rise exceeds 0.75 in one year, repeat the test in one month. If the retest confirms the 0.75 rise, this is a red flag. Your doctor may want to put you on an antibiotic, such as Cipro, for one month to rule out an infection (prostatitis) as a possible cause. If your PSA continues at that level, or moves higher, talk with your urologist about moving to Step 3 in this process – *even if your PSA is within the normal range.*

Example: Say your PSA was 1.5 last year. This year it measures 2.3 (i.e. a greater than 0.75 rise). You retest one month later and the 2.3 is confirmed. Your doctor prescribes Cipro for one month in order to rule out infection as the cause. Retesting one month later confirms the 2.3 reading. You should move to Step 3 – even though your PSA is still within the normal range of 0 - 4.0.

Don't rely on your doctor to raise a red flag on this important measurement. You need to monitor your own PSA velocity. Too often, doctors don't express concern until your PSA level approaches or exceeds the upper limit of the normal range (0 to 4.0). Most labs will automatically flag a number that is higher than 4.0, but they won't tell you if your PSA velocity is dangerously high. Many experts feel that PSA velocity is much more important than the absolute number.

Here is a note I received from one of our BOB members who happens to have chosen an excellent primary care physician:

I've been tracking my PSA for 10 years. It started at 1.0 and was slowly going up each year. Last year it jumped from 1.9 to 2.4. A repeat PSA test resulted in a 2.7 reading. My family doctor, who was giving me my annual physical – not a urologist – knew my family history. My father had passed due to prostate cancer. My mother passed due to breast cancer. He thought that it would be wise for me to get an ultrasound test. He said he'd seen other patients who had aggressive cancers with a PSA at 2.4. The ultrasound was a little "suspicious."

He then did a biopsy which showed cancer. I feel really blessed to have caught this cancer as early as we did. Now I plan to forget about dying from prostate cancer.

PSA is a Relative Indicator

PSA is not an absolute indicator of the presence of cancer. A high PSA doesn't mean you *have* cancer and a low PSA doesn't mean that you *don't*. However, there's a higher probability that you *have* prostate cancer with higher PSA than with low. Equally important is the fact that rapidly rising PSA, *even within the normal range,* can indicate abnormal cell activity and possibly be an early warning of cancer. Some doctors will call attention to this change in PSA within the normal range, but sadly most won't. Therefore, it's up to *you* to be vigilant and to closely monitor your own PSA. Again, remember that this disease is curable if you catch it early.

> *Tip: Always ask your doctor for your PSA results. Don't rely solely on a comment that "everything is fine." Keep a file on your PSA measurements. Track them carefully year after year. Plot them on a graph if possible. If a rise of more than 0.75 ng/mL is observed, even if the number is within the normal range, see your urologist.*

To complicate matters further, recent studies reported in the *Journal of Urology* have shown that about 25 percent of men with PSAs in the upper end (2.5 to 4.0) of the normal range do in fact, have early stage prostate cancer. For this reason, we can expect the top of the "normal" PSA range to be adjusted downward sometime in the future.

There's another important reason for finding the cancer at this early stage: It's been demonstrated that *cure rates* for patients with lower PSAs are better than for patients with higher PSAs, regardless of the treatment option chosen.

Don't Panic at A Single High Reading

There can be several reasons for an abnormally high PSA reading. They include:

1. Prostate infection
2. BPH or benign prostatic hyperplasia, a benign condition

245

3. Laboratory error
4. Any stimulation of the prostate gland

An article in the *Journal of Laboratory Medicine* quantified some of the non-cancer causes for elevated PSA:

Condition/Manipulation	Effect on PSA Increase	Persists
Acute bacterial prostatitis	5-7 fold	6 weeks
Acute urinary retention	5-7 fold	6 weeks
Bicycle or horseback riding	0-3 fold	1 week
Prostate biopsy	Very Variable	6 weeks
Prostate massage	Variable	6 weeks
Ejaculation	Variable	3 days
TURP (transurethral resection of the prostate)	Very Variable	6 weeks

DRE Also Affects PSA Results

A different study added the digital rectal exam to the above list. A DRE performed within 72 hours prior to drawing blood for PSA can cause elevated readings. Many physicians do not know this: Blood should *always* be drawn *before* the DRE is performed. Stimulation of the prostate by DRE will most likely cause PSA to be elevated.

The bottom line is that any activity that might stimulate the prostate gland should be avoided for several days before a PSA blood test is conducted. Many doctors are surprisingly unaware of this fact, or otherwise fail to communicate this information to their patients. I have spoken with numerous men who reported their doctors typically do the digital rectal examination just *before* blood is drawn for the PSA test. Many of these men reported erroneously high readings when the test results came in.

Men often suffer needless anxiety for the several days it takes for the repeat blood test and PSA measurement, only to find out that the elevated reading was a false alarm.

Tip: Be sure to "rest" your prostate for at least four days prior to having blood drawn for a PSA test. No sex; no DRE; no bike rides; no prostate massage; etc.

Lab Errors

Laboratory mistakes are not uncommon. PSA tests, although somewhat automated, are conducted by human beings, and we humans make mistakes, and even automated lab equipment breaks down. Despite the best of intentions, occasional errors occur, and they can result in false readings.

Tip: At the first sign of an abnormal PSA reading, repeat the test. And be sure to abstain from activities that might stimulate the prostate gland for four days before the repeat blood test.

Even if a repeat test confirms the higher reading, it's still not necessarily cause for alarm. There are several non-cancer possibilities that need to be ruled out before proceeding to the imaging and biopsy steps.

Many men have suffered and died from prostate cancer because their doctor didn't measure their PSA, or he/she measured it, but didn't pay attention to the results.

It's impossible to track your PSA if your doctor isn't submitting blood samples to a laboratory for this measurement. Also, not all doctors do a PSA test during the annual physical examination. Make sure your doctor does.

PSA Is Only A *Relative* Indicator

According to *Healthday News*, more than a million prostate biopsies are performed each year. Of these, only 25 percent test positive for cancer, but another 25 percent have false *negative* findings, which means the test comes back negative even though it's later found that the patient does have cancer.

This is changing as newer imaging technologies are greatly improving the 30-year-old "blind" biopsy technology, which is in wide use today. This is discussed in Step 3.

Another important point: researchers found a high PSA level in relation to the size of the prostate was an indicator for prostate cancer even if the first biopsy comes back negative, providing a new clue as to whether a repeat biopsy is justified.

This is just one more reminder that one must take several issues into consideration when looking for prostate cancer (PSA, DRE, PSA velocity, prostate size). And not all doctors pay attention to these things. This is one more reason why it's up to the patient to educate himself about this disease for his own protection. The earlier the diagnosis, the better are your chances of a cure and greater are the number of treatment options available to you.

"The earlier the diagnosis, the better are your chances of a cure and greater are the number of treatment options available to you."

Free-PSA

Free-PSA (f-PSA) is a little used, yet reasonably valuable predictor of prostate cancer. F-PSA can be used when there's suspicion of prostate cancer before a biopsy is ordered. This test could be used to provide additional information that may help eliminate unnecessary, expensive, and uncomfortable biopsies, according to a survey conducted by the *Men's Health Network:* "The survey suggests many doctors are not yet taking advantage of the risk-assessment information that the f-PSA test provides about how likely prostatic biopsies are to show cancers in individual cases," said prostate cancer specialist William J. Catalona, M.D., of the Washington University School of Medicine. "That means patients may not have all the information they need to make an informed decision about whether or not to have a biopsy."

Tip: If your PSA is rising, even if not outside the normal range, consider having a free-PSA test in order to predict the likelihood of a positive biopsy. It might help you avoid the cost and discomfort of a needle biopsy.

Free-PSA is generally expressed in percentages. The higher the percentage, the lower the probability one has prostate cancer. If f-PSA is higher than 25 percent the likelihood of prostate cancer is less than 8 percent. If f-PSA is below 10 percent the likelihood of cancer is greater than 50 percent.

The following table shows how PSA and f-PSA relate to the probability of one's having prostate cancer. As you can see, when both are used together, the predictability improves. In my case, I had a PSA of 7.9, which indicated a 25 percent probability. A f-PSA of 7 percent predicted a better than 56 percent chance of my having prostate cancer. You may recall that I had two previous biopsies with negative results. I wasn't anxious to have a third. However, when the f-PSA results came in, I agreed to the biopsy, which ultimately proved to be positive.

PSA	Probability of Cancer
0-2 ng/mL	1%
2-4	15%
4-10	25%
>10	>50%

% f-PSA	Probability of Cancer
0-10	56%
10-15	28%
15-20	20%
20-25	16%
>25	8%

This was originally presented in the *Journal of the American Medical Association*, JAMA 279:1543, 1998

Digital Rectal Exam (DRE)

The DRE, in conjunction with the PSA test is a valuable tool in helping to detect prostate cancer. Because PSA is a relative indicator, we can't rely on PSA alone to tell us if cancer is growing in the prostate.

Approximately one out of seven men diagnosed with prostate cancer has a PSA in the normal range. Many more men with "normal"

PSAs have undiagnosed prostate cancer. Studies have also shown that one out of four men whose PSA is in the top half of the "normal" range has prostate cancer.

The DRE is a simple, quick and painless test performed in the doctor's office. Details of the DRE are discussed in previous chapters. Compared to the horrors of prostate cancer, this simple test is a "piece of cake." Yet many men avoid it because the thought of it makes them uncomfortable.

Although it's possible to have prostate cancer with normal DRE and PSA in the 0 to 4.0 range, it's likely that one of these two measurements will signal the presence of prostate cancer if it is there.

And remember, *any activity that might stimulate the prostate gland should be avoided for several days before blood is drawn for PSA test.* This includes the DRE.

3. Have Multi-parametric MRI Imaging if PSA is Rising

I covered this subject quite extensively in Chapter 17 when discussing new diagnostic tools and the evolution of prostate cancer testing and detection.

With today's technology, I can't imagine jumping to the invasive and uncomfortable biopsy step without doing a multiparametric MRI – preferably 3-Tesla – to determine if there are any suspicious areas within my prostate *and* also knowing my PI-RADS assessment.

If you have rising PSA, suggesting the possibility of prostate cancer activity, it would be to your great advantage to find a medical center that can perform a 3-Tesla multi-parametric MRI of your prostate. This could tell you a) if there are any suspicious lesions present, and b) if a prostate biopsy is needed at all.

By using mp-MRI imaging you have a significantly greater chance of finding cancer if it's there and providing important information that can be used if a biopsy is ordered.

4. Manage Your Biopsy Test if Above Steps Lead to a Decision to Schedule a Biopsy

If the mp-MRI shows suspicious lesion(s) talk with your doctor about scheduling a biopsy, but on *your* terms.

Have an MRI-Guided Biopsy

As discussed in previous chapters, the MRI-guided biopsy is the latest technology and it provides the best opportunity of finding cancer by targeting suspicious lesions identified by MRI, rather than randomly sampling the prostate using 30-plus-year-old blind biopsy technology. Both the MRI fusion/ultrasound guided biopsy, or the in-bore MRI guided biopsy are excellent choices.

Insist on Local Anesthesia

Biopsies do *not* have to be painful. Many urologists don't even suggest using local anesthesia. I suspect that's because waiting for the patient to "numb-up" slows things down, and fewer patients can be biopsied per hour if anesthesia is used. Keep in mind, the urologist doesn't feel any pain during the procedure.

Any patient who's about to undergo a prostate biopsy should ask for local anesthesia. Why experience the pain and discomfort of a biopsy when you don't have to?

There are several options available to minimize or eliminate discomfort from the biopsy. One study conducted in 2015 and reported in *Urology Annals* compared three anesthesia techniques: 1) Periprostatic nerve block injection using lidocaine, 2) Intra-rectal lidocaine gel and 3) Pudendal nerve block injection using lidocaine. Researchers determined that while all three provided effective pain elimination, the periprostatic nerve block was the best at pain control.

There are other options available to patients to manage pain during prostate biopsy. All generally work well at providing comfort during this procedure.

If your urologist doesn't offer the option of pain management for the biopsy test – especially for a 12- to 24-sample biopsy – I'd recommend finding a new urologist.

Take Steps to Prevent Infection from Biopsy

Unfortunately, about 5 percent of patients who undergo transrectal biopsies experience infections, including dangerous sepsis, with up to 3 percent requiring hospitalization. The reason for this is that the standard antibiotic given to patients prior to biopsy is Ciprofloxacin (Cipro). While Cipro is generally an excellent medication in a class of drugs called quinolone antibiotics, used to prevent and treat bacterial infections, a small percentage of patients have bacteria in their intestines that are quinolone resistant, which means Cipro may not prevent an infection.

A simple and inexpensive Culture and Sensitivity (C&S) test involves taking a swab of the rectal area and analyzing it for quinolone resistance. If the bacteria in your gut is quinolone resistant, your doctor can prescribe an alternative antibiotic, such as Doxycycline or Bactrim.

Sadly, this simple low-cost C&S test is not routinely performed at most institutions today, though it is gaining in popularity and use.

An alternative to the C&S test would be to ask your doctor to consider combining Cipro with Ceftriaxone along with needle washing with isopropyl alcohol. A 2018 study published in *Renal and Urology News* (see appendix), showed this technique to dramatically reduce infection rates.

Another alternative is to have the biopsy done through the perineum (space between scrotum and anus), as this prevents infection from fecal matter getting into the bloodstream. While not commonly done, this technique has been used over the years with much success in controlling infection. *Northwell Health* published an article in 2018 on a newly developed 15-minute, transperineal biopsy that can be performed in an outpatient setting under local anesthesia using standard rectal ultrasound (see appendix).

Biopsy the 'Old-fashioned' Way

If for some reason you don't have access to the latest MRI-guided biopsy technology and you'll be having your biopsy done the "old fashioned" way, you can still manage your biopsy.

The typical prostate biopsy involves imaging the prostate using a rectally inserted ultrasound tube, along with a device that contains a spring-loaded hollow needle to take prostate tissue samples. The ultrasound provides an image of the prostate that helps the doctor guide the needle. When the needle is properly positioned, the doctor "pulls the trigger," and the hollow needle passes through the rectal wall and into the prostate gland where it removes a core sample of tissue.

The more samples taken, the better your chances of finding cancer if it's there. A study by Robert Bahnson, Chief of Urology at Ohio State University, indicated that one in seven prostate cancers is missed with a six-sample biopsy. You should insist on a minimum of 12 biopsy samples.

My first two negative biopsies were six core samples each. My third biopsy involved eight core samples and two of them were found to be cancerous. I truly believe that, had I insisted on a minimum 12 samples the first time, my cancer would have been diagnosed three years sooner, and I would have been spared two additional biopsy tests.

No one ever wants to hear those awful words, "you have cancer," but if it *is* going to happen, it's unquestionably in your best interest to *find it early*. Early detection is critically important and will greatly influence the likelihood of a cure. In other words, *proper sampling and early diagnosis could conceivably represent the difference between life and death.* At the very least, early diagnosis can have significant impact on the *quality of life* following treatment, as early treatment options tend to be "kinder and gentler" than those used for advanced cancers.

Tip: Insist on a minimum of 12 biopsy samples to ensure the cancer is found at the earliest possible stage.

There's an additional benefit to taking a larger number of biopsy samples. If the results come back negative, you can have a greater degree of confidence that there really *is* no cancer in your prostate. In my case, being an engineer familiar with the statistical inaccuracies associated with inadequate sampling, I suspected the cancer was there, even though the first two biopsy reports were negative. I didn't know at the time, however, that I could have requested, or rather *insisted*, on 12, 16, or even 24 samples. As a result, the cancer had an additional two years to grow inside my body, and possibly even migrate to places outside the prostate. I wish *this* book had been available to me back then!

5. Get a Second Opinion on Your Biopsy Results

I can't overemphasize the importance of this step. When you finish reading this section, you'll understand why I feel this way.

Gleason Score is Key

Your Gleason score is probably the most important factor in staging your cancer. It will have a major impact on whether or not you're a candidate for active surveillance, as well as which of the treatment options might work for you.

Your Gleason score will also be a major influence on the need for any adjunct treatments, such as androgen deprivation (hormonal) therapy.

As you know from an earlier chapter the Gleason score is determined by a pathologist evaluating prostate tissue samples under a microscope and looking for five different cell patterns ranging from normal, well-differentiated cells all the way to significantly fused, amorphous cell patterns. He/she then takes the two most predominant patterns and adds them together, putting the most dominant cell-pattern first. This becomes your Gleason score.

While it may sound simple and straight forward, it's not. The process is subjective at best, and errors are frequently made.

'How Doctors Think'

Over the past several years, I've heard from dozens of men who've read my book and took my advice on seeking a second opinion on their biopsy slides, only to learn that the initial reading was incorrect.

How do we know the second reading is correct? If the second reading is done by one of the premier pathology labs at a highly respected medical center – such as Dr. Jonathan Epstein at Johns Hopkins – then you know it's an accurate result that can be used for determining a treatment plan. I've provided a list of some of the premier pathology labs in the appendix.

I recently read the book, *How Doctors Think*, by Jerome Groopman, M.D., of Harvard Medical School. The book reviews Dr. Groopman's experiences both as an oncologist and as a patient. If you ever doubt the importance of seeking a second opinion on medical matters – especially biopsy slides – read this book.

My assessment of the theme of his book is that doctors are human beings and human beings make mistakes. *The patient should become his own advocate, do his research, challenge conclusions and always ask questions.* That is also the theme of this book.

Using radiology as an example, Dr. Groopman notes that in one study at Michigan State University radiologists disagreed among themselves 20 percent of the time! And the same radiologists contradict their earlier analyses 5 to 10 percent of the time.

In another study involving screening mammograms of 148 women, "the fraction of patients actually having cancer who were correctly diagnosed varied from 59 to 100 percent, and the fraction of patients *without* disease who were correctly diagnosed as normal ranged from 35 to 98 percent. Overall, the accuracy rate varied from 73 to 97 percent."

Results from a variety of radiological procedures were summarized by Ehsan Samei of the Advanced Imaging Laboratories at Duke University Medical Center. He concluded that:

> *"Currently, the average diagnostic error in interpreting medical images is in the 20 to 30 percent range. These errors, being either of the false-negative or false-positive type, have significant impact on patient care."*

The same kind of variability can be found in reading biopsy slides, according to Dr. Groopman:

"There can be significant differences in how different pathologists assess the same biopsy."

A Blemish or Cancer

In a March 18, 2017, syndicated *Annie's Mailbox* newspaper article, a patient wrote about his primary care physician of 40 years repeatedly ignoring a half-dollar sized lesion on his arm, "which the doctor covered with a blood pressure cuff every time I saw him."

This same doctor, when asked about a never-healing sore on the patient's forehead, said it was nothing but "a blemish." When a friend insisted he see a dermatologist for a second opinion, he discovered he had a melanoma on his arm and a basal cell carcinoma on his forehead.

No Bladder Cancer

A couple of years ago a gentleman who was treated with external beam radiation for prostate cancer sent me the following email:

I was treated with radiation for prostate cancer four years ago at the age of 65. Last August, because of blood in my urine I went to my urologist and after testing was recommended for a biopsy.

They diagnosed me with invasive bladder cancer. My urologist said it was aggressive but treatable.

Based on your recommendation, I decided to seek a second opinion from Johns Hopkins. They suggested it may not be cancer but something that mimics it called pseudo-neoplastic legions. Upon learning that I was treated with radiation therapy, it reinforced their conclusions. Johns Hopkins suggested I send my slides to Cedars Sinai and Memorial Sloan Kettering. They were both in agreement with

Johns Hopkins. What a relief! I had a follow-up biopsy, and this time there was no evidence of any cancer at all and this was confirmed by Johns Hopkins.

I was encouraged to write to you after reading the December BOB Tales newsletter in regard to the importance of getting second opinions. There appears to be a relationship between radiation and inflammation that can occur afterwards that mimics cancer that most pathologist aren't aware of.

Thank you Brotherhood of the Balloon. If it weren't for your encouragement to get a second opinion, I would have been treated for bladder cancer for no reason at all.

Prostate Cancer Examples

Gleason Score Increased: One gentleman who read the first edition of my book was diagnosed with Gleason 3+4=7 prostate cancer. He decided to follow my suggestion and have his biopsy slides examined by one of the premier labs listed in the appendix.

The results were quite shocking: Gleason 5+5=10! The good news is this individual was properly treated for a much more advanced prostate cancer. In all likelihood, his treatment for Gleason 3+4 cancer would have been much less aggressive, leaving him with a significantly greater chance of a recurrence. Today, several years later, his PSA is 0.4 and he's enjoying life to the fullest.

Gleason Score Decreased: Here's an email I received from another patient who followed my advice

First of all, I want to extend much thanks to you for recommending a second opinion on my biopsy slides. I did so and as a result, my Gleason score was reduced from 3+4=7 to 3+3=6 and my core volume reduced from 15 percent to 5 percent. Per NCCN, using this information, I would now be considered in the very low-risk category with ALL of the following criteria being met:

- *T1c non-palpable - yes*
- *PSA < 10 ng/mL - yes, latest test reduced from 4.5 to 3.3*

- *PSA density < 0.15 - yes, mine .09 per MRI*
- *Gleason score ≤ 6 - mine now 3+3=6, reduced from 3+4= 7*
- *Cores with cancer ≤2 - mine 1*
- *Less than 50 percent in core - yes, mine reduced from 15 percent to 5 percent*

According to NCCN, people in the very low risk category with life expectancy less than 20 years, active surveillance is a very good option. This is what I plan to do after I fire my urologist. To the very end, he refused to send the slides for a second opinion; he told me if I want it that I should do so myself.

No Cancer at All! – Example 1: A gentleman who was diagnosed with prostate cancer was scheduled for a radical prostatectomy. He read my book, got a second opinion and learned he didn't have prostate cancer. He was deliriously happy with this good news and posted the following review of my first book on Amazon:

Always get a second opinion on your diagnosis. April 6, 2007

In January of 2007, at the age of 55, I was diagnosed with prostate cancer. My urologist wanted to operate within two weeks. After finding Bob Marckini's book, "You Can Beat Prostate Cancer and You Don't Need Surgery to Do It," I read it from cover to cover and took his advice. I had my slides reviewed by another pathologist. The results conflicted with the original report, so I sent the slides to Dr. Jonathan Epstein at Johns Hopkins, who is recommended in Bob's book. He stated that I needed another biopsy to be certain, since he could not say that it definitely was cancer. After having the second biopsy... the results came back that I did not have prostate cancer. Had I not read this book I may very well have had needless surgery. This is definitely a "Must Read" for every man diagnosed with prostate cancer. Don't leave your life in the hands of one doctor. Always do your homework and make sure it includes this book.

No Cancer at All! – Example 2: Another gentleman who had been diagnosed with prostate cancer was encouraged by his urologist to have DaVinci laparoscopic robotic surgery. The patient did his homework and narrowed his choices to either DaVinci surgery or proton therapy.

He contacted Loma Linda University Cancer Center for information about proton therapy and they sent him a packet of material, which included a copy of my book. He read the book, followed my suggestions on getting a second opinion on his pathology slides, and discovered that he didn't have prostate cancer! Greatly relieved, he posted a review of my first book on Amazon:

> ### *If you have questions about prostate cancer treatments read this book!*
>
> *If you have been diagnosed with prostate cancer, know or love someone who has, or have concerns about prostate cancer due to a family history, you must read Bob Marckini's book. It is an absolute wealth of information written by an intelligent, inquisitive engineer and spelled out in laymen's terms that anyone can understand. You'll know what questions to ask and be much better informed about the answers you are or are not receiving. As a resource tool alone, it is a treasure for where to find additional information. The writer admits to a bias for proton treatment and for good reason. Read his book and you'll understand why. I did and was about to make a decision between robotic-assisted surgery and proton treatment. I was leaning heavily toward proton treatment when I received a phone call that changed everything.*
>
> *Because of the advice in Bob's book I understood the pathology report on my biopsy slides was subjective and should be read by two different laboratories. One of the many resources in the book was a list of a few premier labs in the country. I took this advice and sent my slides off just to confirm if the cancer was any worse, or better than indicated on the first report. The call I received was from Dr. Epstein, the Director of Surgical Pathology at Johns Hopkins, telling me "you do not have cancer." What I do have is an amended pathology report and a letter of apology from the first*

pathologist. Read the book, question everything, question everyone and then act on it. Whatever course of treatment you select, you'll have the confidence and conviction you're making an informed decision that you can live with.

Finding Out When it Was Too Late: One gentleman who lives in my hometown was diagnosed with prostate cancer. He took his urologist's advice and had his prostate removed surgically. Following surgery, when his prostate was dissected and examined by a pathologist, no cancer was found!

In all likelihood, a second opinion on his biopsy slides would have shown no cancer, which means the surgery and subsequent life-altering side effects could have been avoided.

Examples like these are rare, but they do happen. Often the second opinion confirms the first reading, but it's not uncommon for the second opinion to be different from the first, resulting in better information on which to base the best treatment option.

Summary

It's rare when the second opinion is significantly different from the first, but it's not rare for one of the premier pathology labs to differ from the initial pathology reading. I have seen many cases where a 3+3 was found to be a 3+4 or a 4+3. I have also seen cases where a 4+4 was found to be a 3+4 or a 3+3.

These differences are important and can often mean the difference between choosing a simple treatment for early-stage disease – including active surveillance – or aggressive, invasive, radical therapies for advanced disease.

Bottom line: The reading of pathology slides is subjective at best. It's common for two pathologists to report different Gleason scores when prostate cancer is diagnosed. It's important to know the "true" score so your treatment protocol can be properly designed. Under-treating can result in a recurrence, and over-treating could result in damaging quality-of-life issues.

It's always wise to get a second opinion on your biopsy results from a reputable pathology lab.

"It's always wise to get a second opinion on your biopsy results from a reputable pathology lab."

6. Evaluate All Treatment Options

If you're diagnosed with prostate cancer don't rely on the first recommendation made by your urologist. Unless you're too old or too weak to handle the trauma, he/she will most likely recommend surgery. Remember, urologists are surgeons, and for years, the "gold standard" for prostate cancer treatment has been surgery. Some of us have come to believe that surgery should be called "the *old* standard." There are non-invasive treatment options that offer comparable cure rates without the trauma, blood loss, side effects, or recovery time of surgery.

Tip: Examine all the treatment options and choose the right one for you. Don't let your physician make that decision for you.

Learn about the male anatomy and the location and function of the prostate. Learn everything you can about each of the treatment options you're considering.

If you're considering a radical prostatectomy, learn how the procedure is done. Evaluate all other non-invasive options before choosing surgery. Remember *you* are the one on the receiving end of the scalpel.

If your cancer stage is anything other than early stage, consider having a bone scan. This important test will help determine if the cancer has metastasized, i.e. traveled to distant parts of your body. Once you've ruled out metastasis, your options are many. Proton treatment was best for me. It may not be for you. Others have been successfully treated by the other options listed in earlier chapters.

Put together your own decision matrix. Assign the most weight to those factors which are most important to you. Perhaps taking time away from family and work isn't feasible. This could rule out proton treatment – unless you live near one of the treatment centers and can continue your normal work routine while in treatment.

Perhaps the minimal hospital stay of brachytherapy, combined with quick recovery, is most important to you, even if certain side effects have a higher probability of occurring. Or perhaps you may feel strongly about having the gland with the cancer removed from your body as soon as possible, and thus prefer the oldest method, surgery.

Most newly diagnosed patients have relatively early stage disease, which means you don't have to rush into treatment. You have time to do your due diligence and you owe it to yourself to learn about all the treatment options.

I've spoken with many men who regretted their treatment decision and wished they had done more homework when they were first diagnosed. If you're reading this book, you're doing just that.

NCCN Prostate Cancer Treatment Guidelines

The National Comprehensive Care Network (NCCN) is a highly respected association of 21 cancer treatment centers. Their treatment guidelines should be considered – not blindly followed – when making a treatment decision. The following NCCN guidelines are adapted from Mohler J, et al. NCCN Clinical Practice Guidelines in Oncology: Prostate Cancer. Journal of NCCN. 2010;8:162-200.43:

Risk Group: Very Low
- Stage T1c
- PSA less than 10 ng/mL
- Gleason score 6 or less and not more than two cores with cancer
- Less than 50 percent of core involved with cancer
- PSA density less than 0.15

Newly diagnosed cases: 15 percent
NCCN recommendation:
- Active surveillance when life expectancy is less than 20 years.

Risk Group: Low
- Stage T1c or T2a and
- PSA less than 10 ng/mL and
- Gleason score less than 6

Newly diagnosed cases: About 35 percent
NCCN recommendation:

262

- Active surveillance when life expectancy is less than 10 years.
- Active surveillance, surgery or radiation when life expectancy is more than 10 years.

Risk Group: Intermediate
- Stage T2b-T2c or
- PSA 10 to 20 ng/mL or
- Gleason score 7

Newly diagnosed cases: About 40 percent
NCCN recommendation:
- Active surveillance or external radiation with/without hormonal therapy, with/without brachytherapy or surgery if life expectancy is less than 10 years.
- Surgery or external radiation with/without hormonal therapy, with/without brachytherapy if life expectancy is 10 or more years.

Risk Group: High
- Stage T3a or
- PSA 20 ng/mL or higher or
- Gleason score 8 or higher

Newly diagnosed cases: About 10 percent
NCCN recommendation:
- Surgery or radiation plus hormonal therapy.

7. Talk With Men Who Have Been Through Each Option You Are Considering

Prostate cancer is slow growing. It took years for it to grow to the point where it was detected in your body. In most cases, you don't have to make a treatment decision today, this week, or even this month. Take the time to do your research. Buy and read the best books on the subject. Research the Internet. And, above all, *talk with several men who have had each of the treatments you're considering.*

Remember, most books on this subject are written by doctors or researchers who haven't been through the treatment. Only someone who's been through it can truly relate to you his personal experience.

Make up your own list of questions for these former patients representing each treatment option.

Include questions such as these:

Why did you choose surgery (or brachytherapy, or external beam radiation etc.)? Did you do extensive research? Or did you just accept your urologist's recommendation?

Did you consider any other treatment option? If so, why did you disregard them?

What was your experience of the treatment you chose? Was it positive? Was there any pain, blood loss, or complications?

What short-term side effects did you experience? How long did they last?

What long-term side effects have you experienced?

Ask specific questions about incontinence. Did you experience any incontinence – bladder control problems? Do you have any leakage today? If so, under what conditions?

Ask specific questions about impotence. Have you experienced any changes in sexual function? Are erections the same today as they were before treatment?

When did you have this procedure done? What was your pretreatment PSA, Gleason score, and T-score? What's your PSA today? (Remember, if he had surgery and the prostate was removed, his PSA should be non-detectable. If he had any other procedure, he still has a prostate, and there is most likely a low level of measurable PSA. It should be dropping or holding steady, if he's reached nadir.)

Would you choose this procedure again? This will tell you a lot about this patient's overall evaluation of the option he chose. Several of the men I talked with told me they felt they made the wrong choice.

What advice do you have for me? We can always learn from another patient's experience. If he chose the same treatment option you're considering, perhaps he can tell you about ways to prepare for your treatment or give you ideas that will make your experience less anxiety filled and even enjoyable. I received numerous helpful suggestions and recommendations from former proton patients.

Can you give me the names and phone numbers of others who have had prostate cancer treatment? *You can never talk with too many former patients.* You'll learn more from them than from doctors, books, or the Internet, *especially if you question them in depth.*

8. Make Your Decision Based on What is Best for *You*

Following is part of an email I received from a justifiably angry patient:

I am 56, and about 17 months ago I was diagnosed with prostate cancer and I had radical surgery. My pretreatment numbers were PSA 14.8 and Gleason 9, with 6 of 12 cores showing cancer. I was classified as a T3.

I learned that my urologist knew about proton therapy and did not tell me. He told me I was not a candidate for seeds. He led me to believe that my cancer was contained, and the information he gave me on standard radiation scared me to death.

One of my main fears about surgery was the potential loss of sexual function. My urologist told me that he would only remove one nerve bundle and I should retain my sexual function.

Months after my robotic surgery I have zero sexual function, and I learned that with my high numbers the chance of a recurrence following surgery was very high.

A few months after surgery my PSA was 0.4. Following surgery, it's supposed to be non-detectable. I was then told I needed to have radiation for salvage treatment. With this news I became depressed and began a search for other treatments. I

265

found one paragraph about proton treatment in Dr Katz's "Guide to Prostate health." My first response was, "What is this? And why wasn't I told about it?"

In October-November 2008, I received 38 rounds of proton, 8 rounds of chemo, and two Lupron shots. My radiation oncologist told me that with my pretreatment cancer stage, I should never have had surgery because the likelihood the cancer had escaped the prostate was extremely high.

I am very angry about this and I hope you can share my story with others to help them avoid the mistake I made.

This poor soul had the odds stacked against him at the very beginning. This is an excellent example of why it's so important for the patient to understand this disease, to educate himself about *all* the treatment options, and to get a second or third opinion so he could make an informed decision that is in *his* best interest.

I'm not a physician, so take my next statement with a grain of salt: I cannot rationalize any circumstances under which someone with advanced or aggressive prostate cancer – where the likelihood of extracapsular penetration is high – would choose surgical removal of the prostate. Why? Because this individual would almost certainly be faced with a second, primary treatment to "clean-up" what the surgery missed. So why have two primary treatments (surgery and radiation), when one – radiation alone – would give you the best chance of killing the cancer, both in the gland and in the margins, at the earliest possible time?

The Partin Tables

An extremely useful tool for understanding your cancer's progression is called the Partin Tables or Partin Nomogram. I wasn't aware of this valuable resource when I was diagnosed in late 2000. The original Partin table was developed by Alan Partin MD, PhD at Johns Hopkins in 1993 and has been updated many times since. The Partin tables help doctors and patients determine the potential pathological cancer stage before a treatment decision is made, using the patient's clinical staging: PSA, Gleason score, T-score.

All you need to do is visit the website with the nomogram and enter your PSA, Gleason score and clinical stage (T-score). The nomogram will then determine

- The probability of the cancer being confined to your prostate vs. extending through the prostate capsule into the surrounding tissue;
- The probability your cancer has traveled to the seminal vesicles;
- The probability your cancer has traveled to your lymph nodes.

Doctors today categorize prostate cancer typically at three levels: low, intermediate and high risk. About 70 percent of men diagnosed with prostate cancer are in the low-risk category. This means PSA is less than 10, Gleason score is 3+3=6 and clinical staging is T1 or T2. For men in this category the probability of cancer being confined to the prostate is extremely high – close to 100 percent; there's a zero to 1 percent chance of cancer in the seminal vesicles; and virtually a zero percent chance of cancer in the lymph nodes. The Partin tables will confirm these estimates.

High-risk patients typically have PSAs at 20 or above, Gleason scores in the 8 to 10 range and T-scores at 3 or higher. For patients in this category, the likelihood of cancer moving outside the prostate is extremely high as well as seminal vesicle and lymph node involvement.

Intermediate-risk patients will obviously fall in between, with a wide range of probabilities depending on each patient's clinical staging.

I encourage you to visit the Partin Tables, plug in your own numbers and see what you can learn. The Partin Tables website I typically use can be found at this URL:

https://www.hopkinsmedicine.org/brady-urology-institute/specialties/conditions-and-treatments/prostate-cancer/fighting-prostate-cancer/partin-table.html

There are other sites you may prefer. Just do a search for "Partin Tables" on the Internet. The Partin Tables are a valuable resource and represent one more tool for you to use on your journey.

Leave No Stones Unturned

The better you *truly* understand the treatment options – i.e. the better educated you are – the better will be your treatment decision.

Involve your wife (or significant other), your loved ones, and even your close friends in the decision. Perhaps they'll think of something you haven't considered. Either way, their involvement in your decision will solidify your thinking and commitment to the option you choose. Their involvement will also help erase any doubts you might have as to whether your choice is the best option for you.

If you choose active surveillance or an "alternative" therapy, make sure you continue to monitor your PSA.

Just recently I was contacted by a 59-year-old man who had been diagnosed with mid-stage prostate cancer four years earlier. At that time, he chose to be treated by a naturopath who practiced alternative medicine. The naturopath prescribed a variety of herbs, aromatherapy and environmental medicine. This fellow put himself completely in the hands of this doctor – without monitoring by conventional methods – and four years later, he was faced with shocking news: His PSA had risen to 40, his Gleason score to 9 (5+4), and his clinical stage to T4. Twelve out of 12 biopsy samples were positive for cancer.

This is so sad. I tell this story not to condemn naturopaths and alternative medicine. I've heard stories of excellent results for some people who have chosen alternative options. But whatever path you choose, you should monitor what's going on.

If you follow a spiritual path, pray about the decision. For me this was a most important factor. The more I prayed, the more confident I became in proton therapy as my treatment choice.

In Summary

Too many men – in my opinion – leave their treatment decision up to their doctor. The doctor is typically a urologist; and urologists are typically surgeons. If you're planning to rely heavily on input from the medical profession, then in addition to your urologist, you should involve your primary care physician, a radiation oncologist and a medical oncologist as well as your wife, or significant other, and/or a trusted friend.

9.   Choose from Among the Best Practitioners and Treatment Centers

One gentleman from Canada told me he was considering brachytherapy with a local physician. I asked him how many procedures his doctor had performed. He told me he'd check. When he called back, he told me, "She's done six." I said, "Six per day or per week?" He said, "No, six in total." My response was, "Why not let her practice on someone else?"

There are significant variations in the results being seen by different doctors and hospitals around the world, both in terms of disease-free survival and side effects *for the same procedure.* You owe it to yourself to find out about these differences and to pick a doctor and hospital that have demonstrated the best results. If this means traveling a long distance, then so be it. What's the price of maintaining your potency or bladder control? Certainly, the inconvenience or additional cost of some travel should be worth the benefit of improving your chances of disease-free survival and quality of life after treatment.

If you're considering DaVinci laparoscopic robotic surgery, for example, keep this statistic in mind: Dr. Prasanna Sooriakumaran, a urologist and researcher at the Weill Cornell Medical College in New York, published an article in Bloomberg News reporting that, "Doctors who perform robotic-assisted prostate cancer surgery aren't proficient and able to remove all the malignant cells surrounding the tumor until they have done the procedure more than 1,600 times."

Your primary objective is disease-free survival, and close behind is quality of life after treatment. You have a significantly better chance of achieving both of these goals if you 1) choose a doctor with excellent credentials, reputation and considerable experience, and 2) select a highly ranked treatment facility with a proven track record.

10. Maintain Your Physical And Mental Health

Regardless of the option you choose, your physical and mental health, as well as your attitude can make a huge difference in your treatment experience as well as the results of your treatment. Studies have shown those in better physical health and those with a positive mental attitude statistically have quicker recoveries and higher cure rates. Perhaps this is because the body's immune system is a key factor in preventing regrowth and spread of cancer. Better physical and mental health support a stronger immune system.

If you're not already actively involved in a physical fitness program, begin now. This can be as simple as walking a mile or two a day. Otherwise join a fitness club and work out three or four times a week. Include exercise that will improve cardiovascular fitness, such as jogging, swimming, stationary bike, rowing machine, or stair climber. Of course, you should check with your doctor before engaging in any new physical activity.

Eat a healthy diet. This means minimizing red meats, processed meats, animal fats, and most dairy products. Introduce healthy foods into your diet, such as soy products, fresh fruits, and vegetables. Exercise regularly and maintain proper body weight. Take selected vitamins and supplements to supply your body with nutrients missing from your diet. All these things can help slow or stop the progression of prostate cancer and also help prevent a recurrence.

If you're in a high-risk group (e.g. family history or African American) be extra vigilant about diet, exercise, and monitoring key health measurements.

If you have significant anxiety about your diagnosis and your decision, speak with your priest, minister, or rabbi. Talk with your doctor or a therapist. Perhaps short-term anti-depressant or anti-anxiety medication will help you through the rough spots.

Frequent communications with men who have been successfully treated for prostate cancer can be of great benefit. There are Internet chat rooms, newsletters, man-to-man organizations and support groups of all types available to you. Joining a support group can do much to improve your knowledge, your attitude, and your confidence in the outcome of your treatment for prostate cancer.

Summary

Someone once asked me, "What do you call the guy who graduated at the bottom of his class in medical school?" I said, "I don't know; what do they call him?" The answer, "Doctor."

Not all doctors are created equally. Even some very intelligent doctors can be one-dimensional. They may have great diagnostic skills in certain areas of medicine and be quite uninformed in others. Many diseases and health disorders have obvious telltale signs that any doctor can easily identify. Prostate cancer is *not* one of them.

The best doctors may not be in your community. You owe it to yourself to choose the best family doctor and urologist you can find, even if it means traveling some distance to see them.

Monitoring your own PSA and having an annual DRE will greatly increase your chances of finding the cancer at an early – and thus treatable – stage. The combination of these measurements gives you three tools:

1. **Absolute PSA number**. The top half of the range (2 – 4) is a caution sign. A reading over 4.0 is a red flag.
2. **A rise in PSA** of 0.75 or greater in one year is also a red flag, even if it is within the normal range.
3. **The presence of a lump**, hardness, or other abnormality by DRE is another warning signal.

Doing advanced MRI imaging (3T mp-MRI) and having a biopsy should be discussed with your urologist if:

A. Your PSA is over 4.0, you've ruled out infection as the cause, and a *Free*-PSA test indicates the probability of cancer, or
B. Your PSA is in the 2 to 4 range, you have family history of prostate cancer, and *free*-PSA suggests the probability of cancer, or
C. Your PSA rises 0.75 units or more in one year (even within the normal range) and you've ruled out lab error or infection, or
D. The DRE test detects a lump or hardness in the prostate (regardless of whether PSA is rising or is elevated).

If you and your urologist decide to do a biopsy, consider doing an MRI fusion-guided biopsy or real-time, in-bore MRI-guided biopsy with a minimum of 12 samples, six from each lobe. With early stage prostate cancer, the more samples the easier it is to find.

Ask your doctor for local anesthesia to eliminate the discomfort of the test. He or she can't feel the pain and discomfort – why should you?

If you're diagnosed with prostate cancer, educate yourself on all treatment options. Several books are referenced in the appendix. Explore the Internet. Attend support group meetings in your community. Above all, *interview prostate cancer patients who have completed the treatments you are considering.*

Choose the best option for *you.* And choose from among the best doctors and treatment facilities. This may involve some travel and temporary inconvenience.

Finally, remember that your immune system plays an important role in your body's ability to fight off the growth or spread of cancer, before and after treatment. Give your immune system every possible chance to do its job. Eat a healthy diet; maintain proper body weight; exercise regularly; i.e. take whatever steps are necessary to maintain or improve your physical and mental health.

Prostate cancer is a serious disease, but it doesn't have to be a death sentence. The earlier it's caught, the better your chance of beating it. With the information presented in this book, there's no reason you should have to die of prostate cancer or have your quality of life significantly impacted by the treatment option you choose.

Remember, the most common symptom of prostate cancer is *no symptom at all.* Don't wait for a symptom to appear. If you do, it may be too late to treat with curative intent.

"Remember, the most common symptom of prostate cancer is no symptom at all."

If you follow the advice given in this book, you will undoubtedly die some day – but it will likely not be from prostate cancer.

Most Common Inquiry

As I was drafting this second edition of my book, I received an email from Paul, in Toledo Ohio. It's typical of most of the emails I receive:

> *I am 53 and was diagnosed with Gleason 7 (3+4) prostate cancer on both right (70 percent) and left (30 percent) sides, T2b. I received the bad news two months ago, and I haven't had a good night's sleep since. My PSA is 5.6. I am in good health . . . except for this recent discovery.*
>
> *I've spent the past 8 weeks becoming more and more confused with an overload of info. The surgeons recommend surgery, the radiologists recommend radiation, etc. My search has led me to your website and proton therapy as a real possibility. I would like to know more about this option. Could this be what I've been looking for? How do cure rates compare with surgery and conventional radiation? What about impotence and incontinence? What about rectal irritation and secondary cancers?*
>
> *Please help me – I'm confused and scared.*

That's where I was 19 years ago. This book has been written for men like Paul in Toledo.

Bottom Line

I'm often asked, "What would be your second choice if proton therapy were not available?" My typical knee-jerk response is, "I would not choose surgery of any kind, including the latest forms of robot-guided laparoscopic surgery."

The bottom line for me is this: Why would anyone choose a treatment option that:

- is invasive and painful;
- could result in complications from anesthesia and infection;
- could result in blood loss requiring transfusion;
- requires the wearing of a urethral catheter for days or weeks;
- carries a high probability of impotence and incontinence;

. . . when there are painless, non-invasive treatments available that cure cancer *at least* as well as surgery, and with fewer side effects?

Bradley Hennenfent, M.D., author of *Surviving Prostate Cancer without Surgery* had this to say:

> *"The radical prostatectomy is a sacrifice, not a cure. Its rate of sexual dysfunction is a whopping 100 percent. It leaves all men without semen, with a smaller penis, and with diminished or altered orgasms. The bad news doesn't end there. The operation leaves perhaps 60 percent of its victims impotent, 49 percent with some degree of urinary incontinence, and 16 percent with urinary strictures (scarring and blocking of the urinary passage). All of that – as horrible as it is – might even be worth it to some men if the operation were indeed a lifesaver. Unfortunately, controlled scientific evidence shows that the radical prostatectomy is a failure."*

When I released the first edition of this book, my second choice would have been IMRT. Today, I would consider IMRT. But once again, we're talking about a *second* choice. Proton therapy would always be my first choice.

Remember the carpet bomb vs. smart bomb analogy? Picture a house with a bunch of terrorists that you want to destroy. But it's in a highly populated neighborhood surrounded by other buildings and homes inhabited by innocent people. Would you prefer to destroy the enemy with a carpet bomb that will take out the terrorists' house and with it, neighborhood homes, other buildings and innocent people? Or would you prefer to use a smart bomb that takes out the bad guys' house and does minimal to no damage to the neighborhood?

Now picture that the terrorists' house is your prostate, and the surrounding neighborhood is your bladder, rectum and testes. There's a medical technology that can target the prostate and kill the cancer while doing minimal collateral damage to the "neighborhood." That technology is proton therapy.

If surgery is the "gold standard," for treating prostate cancer, then proton beam radiation therapy is the new "platinum standard."

CHAPTER 19

Impact of Diet and Lifestyle on Prostate Cancer Prevention and Recurrence

"It's choice - not chance - that determines your destiny."
— Jean Nidetch

This topic is so important, I felt it should have its own chapter in this second edition.

Two of the most common questions I'm asked are, "Is there anything I can do to prevent prostate cancer?" and "What can I do to prevent a recurrence of my prostate cancer?"

Medical researchers don't know for sure what causes prostate cancer. But they do know there's a strong genetic component. They also know that diet and lifestyle are contributing factors – sometimes *significant* contributing factors. So short of selecting different parents, there are some things you can do that may help prevent prostate cancer, slow the progression of prostate cancer and help prevent a recurrence.

The Internet is overflowing with diet and lifestyle hints for preventing cancer and other diseases. Much of the information presented has value, but some of it is misleading and even dangerous. I've been following this subject closely for almost 20 years and have distilled the valuable information down to the few, important areas that should be helpful to those of you who are looking for substantive steps you can take to maintain or improve your health, with a focus on cancer in general, and prostate cancer in particular.

Two Important Books

Libraries abound in publications on improving your health, reversing poor health and cancer prevention. Two of the most important books I've read on these subjects are *The China Study*, by T. Colin Campbell and *Anticancer: A New Way of Life*, by David Servan-Schreiber, MD, PhD.

The China Study focuses primarily on the link between the consumption of animal products and chronic illnesses including coronary artery disease, diabetes, breast cancer, prostate cancer and colon cancer. The book concludes that those who eat a predominantly whole food, plant-based diet can avoid or reduce the development of these and other diseases. Data presented in the book overwhelmingly supports the author's hypothesis.

Anticancer: A New Way of Life was written by a physician-scientist who was diagnosed with brain cancer. The author spent months researching scientific data on natural defenses against cancer. In the book, he points out how a poor diet, unhealthy lifestyle and environment increase risk of cancers of all types. The 16-page insert in this book, titled *Anticancer Action*, by itself is worth the price of the book. This insert delineates lifestyle changes, products and foods to avoid, exercise, meditation and thought processes that can improve your health and activate immune cell production. It also lists dozens of foods you can consume to help fight several specific cancers including prostate, brain, lung and breast cancers. And finally, it provides a shopping list for anticancer foods in several categories, such as proteins, grains, fats and vegetables.

There are several important themes in these and other publications I've read on maintaining and improving health, which I will summarize here.

Weigh What You Ought to Weigh

Are you overweight or obese? What's the difference? Men with a body mass index (BMI) below 25 are generally fine. If your BMI is between 25 and 29.9, you're considered overweight; and if it's 30 or higher, you're obese.

How do you determine your BMI? One way is to go to the Internet, search for BMI calculator and plug in your sex, height and weight; the BMI calculator will do the rest.

Another way to determine your BMI is to multiply your weight in pounds by 703, and then divide that number by your height in inches squared. Example: If you are 5' 9" tall, and weigh 212 lbs., your BMI is $(212 \times 703) \div (69 \times 69) = 31.3$ . . . and you're obese.

Why is knowing this important? Because numerous studies have shown a direct connection between obesity and prostate cancer. One study in the U.K. published in *Cancer Research* in 2014 reported that, "men who are overweight or obese are at greater risk of ultimately developing an aggressive form of prostate cancer.

Also, according to an article in the journal, *Cancer* (Volume 109, p 1192), and reported in the *British Journal of Urology International* (Volume 100, p 315) prostate cancer is more likely to metastasize or return after treatment if you're obese. In fact, they reported that, after 10 years, obese men were more than three-times more likely to have developed metastasis and were more than twice as likely to have died of prostate cancer, than their non-obese counterparts.

Bottom line: Obesity is a serious health concern that can affect more than your heart.

Eat a Healthful Diet

The common theme of the above books as well as many of other good books on this subject is that we should avoid, or at the very least, *minimize* our intake of animal products, such as red meat, processed meats, milk and other dairy products. A healthful diet is so important to overall health that we cover this topic every month in our *BOB Tales* newsletter.

The foundation of a healthful diet is to increase our intake of vegetables and fruits, with particular emphasis on cruciferous vegetables (such as broccoli and cauliflower) as well as all dark-green leafy vegetables. We also need to include in our diet richly colored fruits, such as strawberries, blueberries and blackberries.

World Cancer Research Fund recently completed a study involving 26,000 men examining the association between dietary patterns and prostate cancer incidence. The study found that men who chose a vegan diet had a 35 percent reduced risk of prostate cancer. This supports the claims that reducing animal products and increasing vegetables and fruits may be beneficial in preventing prostate cancer.

Other studies show that whole grain breads, cereals, pasta, brown rice, oats, barley, quinoa and other grain products are reported to be beneficial us well.

Healthy protein-rich foods include beans, lentils, chickpeas, split and black-eyed peas and other legumes. These provide both vitamin B and fiber.

Nuts, seeds, olives and avocados provide certain oils that are essential for good nutrition.

The way food is prepared also can enhance your health. Steaming, boiling or baking are generally healthful ways to prepare food.

Foods to Avoid

Foods to avoid include fats and sweets, foods that are high in saturated fat. If you drink milk, it should be skim or low fat. Or better yet, drink soymilk or almond milk. Excessive sugar, alcohol and refined flour also contribute to poor health.

An article in the March 2018 *Colon Cancer Awareness Newsletter* from *Digestive Digest* focused on the role inflammatory diets play in cancer development. Researchers found that processed meat, red meat and organ meat were associated with increased inflammatory markers.

Corn oil contains omega-6 fat, which promoted prostate cancer growth in mice, according to a study reported in *Health24*. The same study showed that fish oil, which contains omega-3 fats shrank prostate cancer tumors in mice. One conclusion reached in this study is that men with early stage prostate cancer who've chosen active surveillance would be wise to avoid a high-fat diet, especially one with corn oil, and to eat a lower-fat diet including omega-3 fats from fish oil.

In a pair of studies published by *Nature Genetics* and *Nature Communications* in 2018, researchers reported that cancer mortality rates in countries with high-fat diets are higher than in countries with low-fat diets. Researchers also concluded from this study that fat consumption is a key environmental trigger for aggressive forms of prostate cancer.

Mediterranean Diet

The two books mentioned above promote a whole food, plant-based diet, which could include a vegetarian or vegan diet. Dr. Charles "Snuffy" Myers, noted prostate cancer expert and prostate cancer survivor, feels the Mediterranean diet is a healthful diet for men concerned about prostate cancer. The Mediterranean diet is based on the traditional eating habits of coastal regions of Southern Italy, Crete and Greece. It emphasizes eating vegetables, legumes, whole grains, fresh fruit, olive oil, nuts and moderate amounts of fish and poultry.

I can't say for sure, which of these diets is best for prostate cancer prevention. But what they have in common is encouraging the consumption of fruits, vegetables, whole grains, legumes and nuts, as well as avoidance of red meat, processed meat, omega-6 fat and dairy products.

Talk with Your Doctor about Vitamins and Supplements

There are differing opinions on taking vitamins and supplements. Some experts, like internist and syndicated columnist Dr. Keith Roach feel that a healthful diet with plenty of fruits and vegetables will provide all the vitamins you need, with the possible exception of vitamin D.

Dr. Roach may be right, but there may not be much harm in taking selective vitamins and supplements just in case your diet isn't providing these things.

On the subject of vitamin D, Dr. Myers has encouraged his patients to monitor their vitamin D levels and to take vitamin D3 as needed to maintain blood levels near the high end of the normal range, because some studies have shown vitamin D to be beneficial in preventing prostate cancer as well as slowing progression of the disease.

Exercise Regularly

Daily physical activity is important for overall good health. A minimum of 30 minutes a day of moderate workout, such as brisk walking, bike riding, swimming or water aerobics is recommended by the World Health Organization. But even leisurely activities, such as yard work have their benefits. A recent study in Taiwan reported that as little as 15 minutes of exercise each day can reduce the risk of death by 14 percent and extend life expectancy by three years compared with those who did no regular exercise.

Reduce Inflammation

Much has been written about the role inflammation plays in the development of cancers of all types, including prostate cancer. Anything you can do to manage/reduce inflammation will strengthen your immune system and help prevent cancer.

Things that can cause inflammation include a traditional western diet high in animal fats and dairy products, smoking cigarettes, leading a sedentary lifestyle and leading a life of stress, anger or depression.

Things that help to reduce inflammation are the opposite of those factors just mentioned: Eating a healthful diet, exercising 30 or more minutes a day, avoiding cigarettes and other pollutants and finding ways to live a more peaceful and serene life. Relaxation techniques such as meditation and yoga may be beneficial here.

My Diet and Lifestyle

I don't claim to have the perfect diet or to be the model for exercise and fitness. However, I do feel that my diet and exercise routines are generally healthful and serve to strengthen my immune system and support the high quality of life that I experience.

Before I was diagnosed with prostate cancer, I ate a reasonably healthful diet and my exercise of choice was running two to four miles three times a week. I have, however, made several changes, particularly after learning from the experts at Loma Linda University

Health, as well as my own research, which included reading the above two books.

My Breakfast, Lunch and Dinner

My breakfast usually consists of three to five servings of fruit (prunes, blueberries, strawberries, blackberries) and hot cereal, such as oatmeal or oat bran with soymilk or almond milk. For additional protein and nutrition, I add whey protein powder and almond flour to my cereal after cooking. These also add flavor and texture to the hot cereal. I drink coffee at breakfast but have given up my morning orange juice as it adds sugar and little nutritional value.

For lunch I usually have a smoothie which is made from an apple, kale, broccoli, frozen strawberries and blueberries, protein powder, goji berries and "Pure Synergy" superfood powder. Despite what you might think, it tastes pretty good.

During the day, I often snack on a handful of nuts (almonds or pistachios) and have two or three cups of green tea. I also drink three or four glasses of water a day.

Dinner most evenings includes a salad with homemade dressing (extra virgin olive oil, apple cider vinegar and spices). My wife and I eat an assortment of homemade soups as entrees, made mostly with fresh vegetables. Chicken, fish and brown rice are on the menu once or twice a week. Several times a week we have fresh vegetables such as broccoli, cauliflower, green beans and legumes (peas, black beans, cannellini beans, kidney beans or lentils). Whenever possible, the fruits and vegetables are organic.

I have eggs and grass-fed red meat occasionally but consume these foods much less often than in the past.

Vitamins and Supplements

I take low-dose aspirin, lycopene, vitamins C, D3, B12 and pomegranate extract. Are all these necessary? Probably not, but it seems to work for me.

Tip: Different from prescription medications, there's no FDA oversite and control over the manufacturing of over-the-counter vitamins and supplements. Be sure to select a quality manufacturer and not just the least expensive option. One of the best suppliers I've found is Life Extension. Vitamins and supplements can be purchased directly from them or through Amazon.

Exercise

A few years ago, I tore the menisci in both knees from running and had to find a different aerobic exercise. My orthopedic doctor, who is a friend, suggested swimming. I've always spent time by the ocean and could swim from point A to point B, but it wasn't very pretty.

So, true to my "recovering engineer" nature, I bought a video on swim training along with goggles, cap and other equipment, and taught myself how to properly swim at a local YMCA. After about three months, I had worked myself up to a mile (36 laps or 72 lengths), which takes me about 50 minutes. I now swim three days a week, 52 weeks a year. I figured recently that since I started swimming for exercise six years ago, I've swum over 1,000 miles!

Another doctor friend who's also a swimmer recently shared with me an article from the July 2019 *Harvard Health Letter*, titled, "Dive into a Swimming Regimen – Lap swimming offers a total-body workout of strengthening, stretching, and aerobic conditioning." The article lists all the benefits of swimming including aerobic activity, improving endurance and cardiovascular health, lowering blood pressure, strengthening all muscle groups, relieving joint pain, increasing flexibility, weight loss, improved balance, sharper thinking, and even meditative benefits from focusing on breathing, which helps reduce stress, anxiety and depression. I truly consider swimming to be the best exercise you can do for your physical and mental health.

In addition to swimming, I work out on the in-between days either at home or at the gym. At home it's sit-ups, push-ups and squats. At the gym I utilize several of the machines, mostly for upper body and legs for a total of about 45-50 minutes.

282

Tip: Find a way to exercise a minimum of three days a week, preferably five or six. Do what works best for you. Experiment. When you find the right exercise routine, you'll know it.

Check with Your Doctor

You should always check with your doctor before making radical changes in your diet, embarking on an exercise program or taking over-the-counter supplements. Supplements are drugs. They can vary in quality and can interact with other medications you may be taking.

Summary

I truly believe in the adage: *You are what you eat.* I'm convinced that with proper diet and lifestyle choices one can prevent cardiovascular disease, diabetes, most cancers, and the recurrence of cancer. It's all about keeping your immune system strong. To strengthen your immune system, you should maintain proper body weight, exercise at least 30 minutes a day, work to maintain a positive mental attitude, and eat a healthful diet.

Strengthen Your Immune System

I learned so much from the extraordinary staff at Loma Linda University Health both during my eight weeks of treatment, as well as the many years of association with them.

In a talk given by Dr. James M. Slater at an Advisory Council meeting, I learned that during our lifetime, dozens of cancers and other diseases infiltrate our bodies. But thankfully, most of them never gain a foothold. The reason? Our immune system fights them off.

So, the message here is: You should do whatever you can to strengthen your immune system. This can help you ward off debilitating diseases throughout your lifetime.

Some of the things you can do to strengthen your immune system include:

- Eat a healthful, balanced diet;
- Weigh what you ought to weigh;
- Exercise regularly;
- Get enough sleep;
- Drink lots of water; and
- Maintain a positive mental attitude.

The Harvard School of Public Health and the Mayo Clinic have linked a positive mental attitude to lowered risk of heart disease and a slowing of the aging process. The American Cancer Society reports that a positive mental attitude improves the immune response. They even go so far as to say that, "Being part of a support group following cancer treatment improves quality of life and enhances patient survival."

Faith and Spirituality

The effect of spirituality on health and the immune system is an area of active research being studied by physicians, psychologists and other professionals. Religious affiliations and spirituality have been shown to enhance whole patient care for patients dealing with potentially life-threatening diseases.

Research has also shown a connection between people's beliefs and their sense of well-being. Positive beliefs, comfort and strength gained from religion, meditation, spirituality and prayer can contribute to well-being, and this can directly benefit your immune system.

I believe that for me and my family, faith and spirituality have played a major role in our health, healing, relationships and happiness.

Final Thoughts

"Choosing to be positive and having a grateful attitude is going to determine how you're going to live your life." – Joel Osteen

Here's an email I received from the daughter of a prostate cancer patient about the first edition of my book:

> *I am full of fear, doubt, optimism, and hope. A month ago, my dad was diagnosed with prostate cancer and my entire world was turned upside down.*
>
> *I was scared and felt like the universe was against him. Shortly after he learned he had prostate cancer a friend gave him your book to let him know there was an option available to him other than surgery. My dad has since spoken with several members of the Brotherhood. Those men are all truly amazing and have been incredibly helpful.*
>
> *Everyone in our family has read your book from cover to cover. My dad begins re-reading it every time he finishes it. In your book you talk about the moment you heard that ominous message from your doctor. You wrote, "I have 'The Big C.' My heart pounded; my mouth went dry; and all the color went out of my world." When I read this part of the book I broke down. This is what happened to me. I walked around every day with this burning in my eyes like I could begin bawling at any time. I'm 24 years old and the thought of losing my dad is earth shattering. I need my dad around to make me laugh till I cry, to be a better person, and to walk me down the aisle next summer. Your book gave him hope that he wouldn't have to face scary surgery, and that there was a better option out there.*
>
> *He has been in communication with the proton center and they have been very helpful. My dad is scheduled for proton therapy thanks to you and your book. I am confident he's going to be fine, that he will be walking me down the aisle on my wedding day, and that he will be with us for a long, long time. God bless you!*

Deb and I have received hundreds of emails and letters like this over the years. This is what keeps us going. It tells us we're on the right path by calming fears and helping people navigate the complexities of the prostate cancer journey.

I hope that after reading this book you realize that, while prostate cancer is something you must take seriously it's highly unlikely to threaten your life or even alter your life in any meaningful way; and that your diagnosis is almost never an emergency requiring urgent action or immediate decisions.

For many with early stage disease, active surveillance or disease monitoring is all that is needed. And for most of the rest, there is plenty of time to study, gather data, and make an informed decision about which of the many treatment options is best for you. A small minority of patients with advanced disease will have to act more promptly, but there's always time for careful analysis, data gathering and decision making.

Your challenge is to take the time to do your due diligence and make the decision that is best for *you*.

My Bias

The title of this book certainly conveys my feelings on the surgical option. If what you've read so far hasn't caused you to take pause at your urologist's recommendation, you may want to read a comprehensive article titled, *Is Robotic Prostate Cancer Surgery Bad Health Advice?* By Bert Vorstman, BSc, MD, MS, FAAP, FRACS, FACS and originally published at https://urologyweb.com on June 10, 2019. Dr. Vorstman is a retired board-certified urological surgeon. While the author focuses on robotic surgery, he also comments extensively on open surgery. If you're seriously considering surgery, you owe it to yourself to read this article.

Not a Death Sentence

Prostate cancer is not a death sentence. If you become your own advocate, properly educate yourself, ask a lot of questions and follow the steps outlined in this book, *you* can take control of *your* diagnosis *and* treatment.

For me this has been a most incredible journey, one I wouldn't change for anything in the world. I was most fortunate to have discovered proton therapy. I'm convinced it cures localized prostate cancer at *least* as well as any other option, with the added benefit of leaving the patient with the best quality of life after treatment.

I wish you good luck, good health and Godspeed in your journey, and I welcome your emails at RMarckini@protonbob.com, with comments, questions and suggestions.

And, remember:

You can beat prostate cancer,
and you don't need surgery to do it.

"Life is not a matter of holding good cards, but of playing a poor hand well."

\- Robert Louis Stevenson

Acknowledgments

Acknowledging people always carries the risk that some will be left out, and I'm sure that's the case here. That said, I would like to take that risk and thank the following people for their help and support: First my daughter, Deb Hickey for her support, encouragement, edits, rewrites and fanatic attention to detail. Deb's husband Mark, a brilliant graphic designer, is responsible for the cover design and most of the graphics in the book. And thank you to my daughter Susie for her prayers and encouragement as I labored over this second edition.

Also thank you to hundreds of members of the Brotherhood of the Balloon whose watchful eyes seem to find every meaningful book, article or Internet reference on prostate cancer prevention, detection, and treatment, and have sent them to me over the years. My library overflows with these publications, many of which have provided valuable information for this book.

Special thanks to the late, Nick DeWolf – a fellow "recovering engineer" – whom I first reached out to through his website 20 years ago. We would later become good friends. His brilliant "Decision Matrix" has appeared in both editions.

Much appreciation goes to Dr. Terry Wepsic for reviewing the manuscript and for his valuable suggestions that have enriched this second edition.

Thank you to all those who reviewed the manuscript and provided endorsements and testimonials. These superb commentaries add much to the book's credibility and value and give readers confidence in the content.

Many thanks to my friend and editor, Bob Hawley who, with great professionalism and expertise, poured over the final manuscript with a "fine tooth comb," greatly improving the final product.

A very special thank you to Loma Linda University Health, where proton therapy was pioneered at great financial risk to the institution. Through their efforts, the technology has been a major success, has grown exponentially worldwide, and hundreds of thousands of patients are the beneficiaries. The support from LLUH to me personally has been unparalleled. Senior management, clinical and administrative staff have opened their doors and hearts to me every step of the way. They have become a second family to me.

A sincere thank you to my friend, Dr. J. Lynn Martell. Without his early recognition of my passion for this subject matter along with his encouragement and support – in so many ways – our organization, *The Brotherhood of the Balloon* might not have survived, and this book might never have seen the light of day.

A huge thank you to my "big brother" Gene for being my teacher and mentor, for smoothing the way for me throughout my life and for his gift of making the prostate cancer journey before me, providing me with the motivation to search for, and find the treatment option that would change my life forever.

I would also like to thank my friend, Joe Bruno for his steadfast interest, support, encouragement, ideas and editorial input.

Most of all, I am indebted to my wife, Pauline, for her tolerance for my long hours at the computer – warming up dinners at 11 pm to allow me to continue writing; for her tolerance and understanding, as every page of my manuscript was taped to the walls of every room in our house – for months; for her many reviews of manuscripts; and for her belief in me and her inspiration which have never wavered.

I apologize to those I've overlooked. There are certainly many more people who have played an important role in my prostate cancer journey.

Appendix A

Terms and Abbreviations

Active Surveillance	Formerly referred to as "watchful waiting," active surveillance is the process of monitoring the cancer without any immediate medical intervention.
Adenocarcinoma	This is the most common cancer of the prostate. It begins in the glandular cells that produce prostatic fluid.
Apoptosis	This refers to programmed cancer cell death following radiation.
Biopsy	This procedure involves the removal of multiple tissue samples from the prostate using a spring-loaded needle. Six to 20 samples are typically taken. Local anesthesia is recommended to minimize discomfort. Some blood is often found in the urine and semen for days or weeks following a prostate biopsy.
Bone Scan	Bone Scan is a 2-Dimensional image of the skeleton using a radioactive tracer. This is a common test to detect cancer that has spread to the bone, a favorite site for prostate cancer to go to.
BPH	Benign Prostatic Hyperplasia. A non-cancerous condition of the prostate gland. It typically refers to an enlarged prostate that may cause a pinching of the urethra and restriction of urine flow. This is a common condition in older men.
Brachytherapy	Seed-implant therapy. Radioactive seeds are implanted in the prostate, destroying cancer by radiating the gland from within. There are two types of brachytherapy, LDR (low dose rate) permanent seed implant, or HDR (high dose rate) temporary seeds that are not left in the patient.

Chest X-Ray	Chest X-Ray (CXR) is a 2-dimensional image of the lung, ribs, and back bone using X-rays. A CXR is commonly used to detect the spread of cancer to the chest area and for screening for other diseases.
Cryosurgery, Cryoablation	Extremely low temperature liquid nitrogen freezing of the prostate and tumor. Becoming more popular as a focal treatment as whole gland cryosurgery often results in erectile dysfunction and incontinence.
CT Scan	Computerized Tomography is a 3-dimensional image of the body using X-rays. CT is a commonly used 3-D imaging tool to help detect cancer that has metastasized (spread) beyond the tissue or organ where it started from. CT is useful when looking for the spread of cancer into the nearby bone and lymph nodes.
DRE	Digital Rectal Examination. A gloved finger is inserted into the rectum to feel the prostate gland to determine if there are any abnormalities.
EBRT	External Beam Radiation Therapy, generally thought to be photon, or X-ray radiotherapy, but it also includes other forms of radiation, including proton.
Free-**PSA (FPSA)**	Refers to the percentage of unbound PSA to bound PSA. The higher the *Free*-PSA percentage, the lower the probability of prostate cancer.
Gleason Score	Refers to the measure of the aggressiveness of the cancer and an indirect predictor of the likelihood the cancer has spread beyond the prostate capsule. Six to 20 tissue samples are taken by needle biopsy and are examined under the microscope. Two areas where cancer is found are graded on a scale of 1 through 5. The two grades are added together to yield the Gleason Score, which ranges from 6 to 10.
HIFU	HIFU (high intensity focused ultrasound) is a procedure that uses high intensity, focused ultrasound to heat and destroy diseased tissue. It is more widely used as a focal treatment.

High-dose Rate Brachytherapy	Seeds are removed after treatment. Usually combined with external beam radiation.
Hormone Therapy	Also known as Hormone Ablation Therapy (HAT) or Androgen Deprivation Therapy (ADT). This treatment, often used in conjunction with other therapies, is intended to shut down the production of male sex hormones (androgens), such as testosterone.
Immuno-therapy	Treatment designed to enhance the immune system's ability to fight cancer
Impotence	Inability to have an erection sufficient for intercourse.
IMPT	Intensity Modulated Proton Therapy. Also known as pencil beam or active beam scanning, an advanced form of proton therapy.
IMRT/IGRT	Intensity Modulated Radiation Therapy (or Image Guided Radiation Therapy), an advanced form of X-ray, or photon, external beam radiation therapy using advanced targeting methods.
Incontinence	Inability to hold urine without leakage. Fecal incontinence is the inability to control bowels.
Libido	Sex drive.
Metastatic Cancer	This is cancer that has spread beyond the prostate to lymph nodes or bones. Cancer that has moved outside the prostate within the prostate bed is not considered metastatic.
Morbidity	In the context of evaluating prostate cancer treatment alternatives, the term "morbidity" refers to side effects. These can be further characterized as Grade 1, 2 or 3 gastrourinary or gastrointestinal morbidity.
MRI	Magnetic Resonance Imaging is a 3-dimensional image of the body using magnets and radio waves that is very different than a CT. Some of our tissues and organs are seen better by a CT, some by MRI, and some by combining both. MRI is useful to detect the spread of cancer in the soft tissues.

Multipara-metric MRI	Mp-MRI is an advanced MRI procedure that provides very precise images of the prostate and can often determine the presence or absence of prostate cancer, or if the cancer is spreading.
PBT	Proton beam therapy or proton treatment
PET Scan	Positron Emission Tomography scans use radioactive materials to determine the presence of tumors. Whole body PET scans are commonly done to detect cancer.
PIN	Prostatic Intraepithelial Neoplasia. This is a pre-cancerous stage of tissue, observed from prostate biopsy, that may become cancerous in the future. Some pathologists do not consider PIN significant.
Prostatitis	A common inflammation or infection of the prostate.
PSA Test	Prostate Specific Antigen Test. This measures the amount of PSA in the blood in billionths of a gram per thousandths of a liter. It is not an absolute indicator of cancer. Prostate cancer may be present at low PSA levels and absent at high PSA levels. PSA is a relative indicator, at best, and should be used along with other measures and observations before any treatment is ordered. PSA is often used as an indicator of cancer recurrence following treatment for prostate cancer.
PSA Velocity	The rate at which PSA is rising, usually expressed in terms of "PSA doubling time."
RP	Radical Prostatectomy or surgical removal of the prostate
SBRT	Stereotactic Body Radiation Therapy. This is a form of external beam radiation therapy, which is highly focused using 3D coordinates to target the exact location of the target volume. Typically, SBRT is delivered in higher doses over a shorter period of time than other radiotherapy options.
Testes, testicles	Housed inside the scrotum. Men's reproductive organs and the primary source of male hormone, testosterone and sperm.

Testosterone	Male hormone or androgen, which is essential for sex drive and fertility.
TRUS	Transrectal Ultrasound. High frequency sound waves are used to determine if there are any abnormalities in the prostate. The TRUS-guided ("blind") biopsy represents the older, less precise, and most common method of determining the presence of prostate cancer.
T-Staging	This typically refers to the size of a nodule within the prostate as determined by digital rectal exam and is also known as clinical staging. There are two staging systems: ABCD and TNM. The TNM is more commonly used today, with the N referring to possible lymph node involvement and M representing distant metastasis.
TURP	TURP: Transurethral Resection of the Prostate. This is surgery to remove tissue obstructing the urethra. The technique involves inserting an instrument called a resectscope into the urethra and is intended to relieve obstruction of urine flow due to enlargement of the prostate.
Ultrasound	An imaging process that creates a picture using high-frequency sound waves. It is usually done transrectally to determine the size of the prostate and to direct the needle used for biopsies.
Urethra	The tube that serves as a conduit for urine and for secretions from the ejaculatory ducts and the prostate.

Appendix B

Proton Patient Testimonials

Terry Wepsic, MD
Diagnosed at age 61 in 2003
Treated at Loma Linda Univ. Cancer Center, Loma Linda, CA

Dr. Wepsic is a physician/pathologist with a specialty in cancer biology and tumor immunology

When I was diagnosed with prostate cancer in 2003 at age 61, as a pathologist, my first inclination was to "cut it out; examine it; and be done with it." But after considering the potential complications of major surgery, I decided the risks were too significant and surgery may also be "overkill" for my early-stage disease.

I considered brachytherapy because it could be done quickly. But, because the seminal vesicles, margins and prostate bed wouldn't be treated with seeds, and I had concerns about side effects due to overlapping radiation, I continued my research.

Fortunately, I found my way to proton therapy at Loma Linda University Cancer Center. I later wrote, in a letter to *The Wall Street Journal,* about my treatment choice:

Proton beam therapy is totally different from any other form of radiation therapy. Energy from the proton is released only when it stops traveling. Eighty-five to 90 percent of the protons go to the target (the prostate). Only 10 percent goes to adjacent tissue. This contrasts with an effective dose of 60 percent for gamma radiation. Protons can be precisely targeted by exact positioning of the patient and the beam. Radiation can include the area surrounding the prostate capsule and the seminal vesicles. These are two areas where tumor spread can occur, even in early stages of disease ... The cure rate for prostate cancer is comparable to all other forms of treatment, but with proton therapy, the side effect profile for erectile dysfunction and incontinence is lower. Many patients have had full post-treatment recovery, including myself.

I'm happy I chose proton treatment and Loma Linda University Cancer Center. The facility is first rate; the people are professional and caring; and the patients were fun to get to know. When I finished my treatment, I remember having separation anxiety, but I wasn't sure if it was from the balloon, the patients, the staff, or the whole enchilada.

Today, I feel well. I'm happy to report I've had no significant side effects and I'd choose proton therapy again and again. It was a wonderful treatment for me, my wonderful wife, and my extended family and friends; we all share a commitment to fully engage in life."

Gary Dilts
Diagnosed at age 68 in 2019
Treated at University of Florida Health Proton Therapy Institute, Jacksonville, FL

"I've had no side effects during or after treatment."

My annual physical uncovered an elevated PSA. My physician said, "Don't worry about it – have it tested again in 90 days." I went home and did my own research online. I found the 2+ point rise in my PSA was a concern, so I got a 4K blood test. That led to a biopsy and my prostate cancer was confirmed.

My urologist was adamant that proton therapy wasn't a solution. He recommended surgery or photon radiation for my stage 2 diagnosis. He wanted to get started right away and suggested traditional radiation with no further testing.

Interestingly, the University of Florida Health Proton Therapy Institute and my oncologist there refused to do any treatment without comprehensive testing. That included a CT scan, two MRIs, a chest X-ray, a bone scan and later, a colonoscopy.

298

The advanced MRI that I had, revealed that my cancer was outside the prostate, but no lymph node involvement. My diagnosis subsequently changed to stage 3B, which required additional considerations including androgen deprivation therapy (ADT). Note: Had I had the recommended traditional photon treatment, I wouldn't have had these additional tests and wouldn't have known the level of cancer I was dealing with.

After my urologist's recommendation, I spent the next 30 days going back and forth between the various treatment options and read everything I could find to make my decision. I found the book, *You Can Beat Prostate Cancer,* by Robert Marckini to be a valuable tool in this process as it broke things down into understandable "patient level language." The book also referred me to several online sources of information that mitigated the negative information regarding proton therapy that the old school medical profession was distributing. I also learned that Robert Marckini founded the "Brotherhood of the Balloon" organization that promotes prostate care and proton therapy and offers a comprehensive website (www.protonbob.com) with a trail of patient testimonials that I found invaluable.

My final decision led me to UFHPTI. My treatment program consisted of 39 daily sessions. We elected to go with a four-month ADT injection that began two months ahead of my treatments. This decision was on the margin given my diagnosis, but viewed to be a good insurance plan that would maximize the effectiveness of my proton stage 3B treatments.

The treatments were administered with a level of precision and professionalism that I've never seen, despite having worked in an industry that demanded extreme levels of quality and process controls. I'm now a year from my final treatment and my PSA remains steady at 0.2. I've had no side effects during or after treatment. The ADT, which was also concluded a year ago, slowed me down; but I've remained active. In fact, I lost five pounds from the exercise and better diet I added to my routine to avoid the expected weight gain from ADT.

I should note that the photon radiation providers followed up with me until the day I began proton treatment, trying to steer me away from proton therapy. I felt like I was being chased by a car dealership that was desperate to close their month with one more sale.

Since my treatment, I've met with many of my friends living in our Florida community who've undergone surgery, photon and proton radiation. Put simply, I haven't found a single person who didn't have an excellent result from proton treatment – and all had no side effects. Conversely, we have friends in our network who've had horrific experiences from surgery and photon radiation, including a surgeon from a prominent hospital who recently had surgery. He's suffering from incontinence and impotence since his treatment and is now undergoing radiation to eliminate the cancer that remained. The pain and discomfort he's experienced has been extreme and far more than he anticipated despite his professional background.

My bottom line: Read everything you can about the various treatment options and be your own advocate. Robert Marckini's book is invaluable and contains the information you need to make an informed decision in this fast-changing cancer treatment environment.

As a final note: I was blessed to have met the husband and wife oncology team, Bill and Nancy Mendenhall at UFHPTI. Nancy was one of the key founders for the facility and spent nearly a decade bringing it to life. She's working on a research project to quantify the success rate proton therapy is providing which will build on the already mounting evidence that proton therapy is truly a breakthrough treatment in cancer care. Her husband, Bill, oversaw my treatment and was available anytime day or night to answer my questions and concerns. What a gift they gave me with my restored health and a new outlook on life!

Finally, my wonderful wife, Randa, was by my side through all the fear, tears and prayers that led me through this process. She never missed a moment of my experience and provided the positive support that kept me going and led me to restored health and a new outlook on life.

Jim Horton
Diagnosed at age 65 in 2015
Treated at Provision Cares Proton Therapy, Knoxville, TN

"Speaking with these men (former proton patients) was a GAME CHANGER. After speaking with about six, my mind was made up."

My prostate cancer experience began with an increasing PSA in October 2014 – it was 5.3. My urologist suggested a biopsy, which resulted in 4 of 12 samples being cancerous. As I expected, my doctor encouraged me to have surgery right away, so he "penciled me in" for removal in just 10 days.

My best buddy had a prostatectomy about a year earlier and he had devastating results. Knowing what he went through, I wasn't willing to take such drastic measures without learning if there were other options available to me. So, I informed my urologist that I needed time to do some of my own research.

Immediately, my wife began searching the Internet. This is how we learned about proton therapy. We contacted three or four proton therapy facilities and quickly settled on Provision in Knoxville, TN. They were professional, friendly and informative.

Still, I was apprehensive because I viewed proton therapy as an "alternative treatment" – I'd never heard of it, and my doctor hadn't even mentioned it. It was imperative I learn more about it from the people who knew it best – men who'd gone through it.

Knowing a little bit about HIPAA regulations, I never expected to be able to speak directly with men who'd undergone proton therapy, but the folks at Provision sent me a list of *dozens.* Speaking with these men was a GAME CHANGER. After speaking with about six, my mind was made up. These men were sincere, open, cooperative, and informative. All of them took as much time as I needed to answer my questions. I had to leave voice mail messages for a few of them and they all returned my call. I became excited to complete my treatment just so I could become an "ambassador" like these guys!

During my treatments, the technicians made sure I understood everything that was going on and that I was comfortable. It still amazes me that the process was so painless and effortless – easier than going to the dentist!

My outcome is better than I could have ever hoped for. I never had a need for adult diapers and there have been no restrictions on my activities. I have slight urgencies to use the bathroom from time to time, but this could be more a product of my age than the proton therapy treatment.

My desire to become a proton ambassador has become a reality and it's a very satisfying experience! In fact, my twin brother was diagnosed with prostate cancer. We served in Vietnam together while in the Army. Over 40 years later, we learned we were in the "second-highest concentration" of spraying of agent orange (thought to cause prostate cancer) in Vietnam. My brother feels blessed that he has me to counsel him on treatment options. He'll begin proton treatment in a few weeks.

Arnd Hallmeyer, MD
Diagnosed at age 57 in 2001
Treated at Loma Linda Univ. Cancer Center, Loma Linda, CA

"The shocking result was a PSA of 436!"

My name is Arnd Hallmeyer. I'm from Berlin, Germany, and work as a physician in the field of occupational medicine. I was 57 when I was diagnosed with prostate cancer. My PSA was 436 and my Gleason score was 5.

In the beginning of my professional life, I worked as a surgery nurse. After I received my medical degree, I became a surgeon.

Over the years, I participated in a few radical prostatectomies and I witnessed some horrible outcomes – impotence, castration, and some patients wearing diapers for the rest of their lives. Because of those experiences, I didn't visit a urologist and I didn't have my PSA checked. I was afraid of ever being faced with the diagnosis of

302

prostate cancer and having to go through the same experience of radical prostate surgery patients. *It seemed better to die than to live life after prostate surgery.*

A few years later, I started having severe bone pain. My wife, Connie, also a physician, and my personal family doctor, became concerned. She started doing some research and told me I had to have a blood test. *The shocking result was a PSA of 436!*

I became deeply depressed, thinking the end of life was near. My father had died tragically at the age of 58 from prostate cancer – it had metastasized to his liver and kidneys. I worried the same was happening to me.

While Connie and I were reluctantly researching prostatectomy surgeons, I had a chance conversation with a well-known radiation oncologist. When I told him about our research he said, "Why are you looking for surgeons? You need Loma Linda." *Loma Linda?* "Is that a medicine or a mystic?" I asked. "Loma Linda is the only place in the world you can be healed with proton therapy," he answered.

I called my daughter, Sigrun, also a physician who worked in a large hospital in Harrisburg, PA. I asked her about proton therapy and Loma Linda. She made some phone calls, did some Internet research, and found her way to Dr. James Slater, "the pioneer of proton therapy."

Although we had some difficulty setting up appointments due to travel, the folks in Loma Linda's International Circle of Care did a great job coordinating things and making me feel at ease. In December 2000, I made my first visit to LLUCC and started treatment in early January. My treatment consisted of protons and photons, as well as hormone blockers, due to my extremely high PSA.

When I came to Loma Linda, everything was foreign to me. I didn't even have experience being a patient. I'd never visited a hospital in my life. I'd also never been to the U.S., and my English was very poor. I had to rent an apartment, a car, and a phone. I also had to shop, cook, and wash my clothes – these things were difficult for me.

What came easily was making friends. Each person I met at the proton center was friendly and helpful. I began to feel like part of a family – not a stranger, not even a patient. I thought, *this must be what that "Make Man Whole" philosophy is all about.* The people at LLUCC were not only treating my disease; they were healing my soul. Throughout my treatment, I made more and more friends – including Bob Marckini and members of *The Brotherhood of the Balloon.* With the help of these people, I was able to adapt to my situation.

I changed my treatment time to early in the morning or late in the evening. This allowed me to attend group outings and hike in the mountains of the San Bernardino Valley. Coming closer to heaven, I found my way back to earth.

I graduated from proton treatment on March 8, 2001. I continued with the hormone blockers for a year. I experienced some hot flashes during that time, but they subsided around January 2002. In September 2002, my PSA was undetectable. I had no pain, just some intermittent rectal bleeding which lasted about a month and then went away on its own.

Nineteen years after treatment, I'm doing very well. My PSA has been steady at 0.1 ng/mL for years, and I have normal bladder and bowel function. I truly believe the best place for prostate cancer healing is in Loma Linda, CA. I've referred countless patients from my own practice to LLUCC and have repeatedly witnessed the transformation of devastated cancer patients into thriving survivors. I've been touched deeply – first personally, and now professionally – and this experience has saved, changed, and inspired my life.

I'm immensely grateful to LLUCC for lighting my path to happiness and fulfillment. I'm now 78 and still able to work full time in my profession as physician manager of two occupational health centers registering typical 60-hour work weeks. I'm the proud grandfather of nine grandchildren.

Because of my experience, I feel I have so much to pass on – so much to teach. I became a member of the LLUCC International Advisory Council and travel frequently to Loma Linda to serve as a voluntary faculty member (professor). And, together with Dr. Jerry Slater and the good people at Loma Linda, one of the best private hospitals in Berlin and many good German friends were able to establish a proton treatment unit in Berlin. It wasn't about making a 1:1 copy of the Loma Linda proton treatment center, but bringing the benefits of proton therapy and the spirit of LLUCC to Europe. It's my deep desire to pay forward what I've been given.

Roger Hutson
Diagnosed at age 65 in 2019
Treated at Mayo Clinic, Rochester, MN; Transferred to Mayo Clinic, Phoenix, AZ

In the spring of 2014, my doctor informed me that my PSA had risen from 3.0 to 4.89 over the previous year. He recommended I see a urologist for additional testing.

I was 60 years old at the time and in relatively good health. I'd never smoked; I was active; I owned two businesses; I'd been married 39 years and was enjoying life with my two grown children and six grandchildren.

I met with a local urologist and a biopsy was performed. I waited a week for the results. Eventually, I was told I had atypical cells in one area of my prostate. The doctor recommended I have another biopsy in six months.

After my second biopsy, I waited two weeks and heard nothing, so I called the urologist's office. I was told he was on vacation and someone else would get back to me. At that point, I didn't have a good feeling about this office.

I decided to get a second opinion at the Mayo Clinic in Rochester, MN. By then it was October 2014. I had a PSA test and a DRE. My PSA had dropped to 3.8, so the plan was to check my PSA again in six months and maybe have an MRI as well.

In June 2015 my PSA was still 3.8 and an MRI showed no evidence of clinically significant cancer. My DRE remained stable. It was recommended I continue to monitor my PSA closely.

In August 2016 my PSA had risen to 5.57. In September 2017 it was 5.78. By June 2018 it was up to 9.05 and I had another MRI that showed no significant change from the previous one. In December 2018 my PSA was down to 7.6 and we scheduled a follow-up six months later.

In July 2019 my PSA was 8.6 and an MRI showed 4 lesions. A biopsy followed. I received a call with the results. I had prostate cancer and my Gleason score was 3 + 4. All I heard was *cancer*. I felt numb. I knew my life was about to change.

My research into treatment options began. I searched the Internet for anything I could find about prostate cancer. Many nights, I stayed up until 3:00 a.m., glued to my computer screen. I found several books on treatment options, a few that mentioned proton beam radiation therapy. A book titled *You Can Beat Prostate Cancer: And You Don't Need Surgery to Do It* by Robert J Marckini caught my attention. I ordered it on Amazon, and it arrived two days later with a handwritten note inside. It read: *Sorry! We're currently out of stock for the book that you ordered from us! However, I've realized that you immediately need the book. Thus, I'm going to send you a used one that I have in my inventory. The book will be a gift from us to you. I hope you will accept it.*

Wow. I realized this wasn't about making money – people really cared!

I read the book in its entirety that day and it was exactly what I needed. I then contacted six members – all former prostate cancer proton patients – of the Brotherhood of the Balloon to learn more about their personal experiences. They were all very encouraging. Some even offered to meet me in person! I was sold on proton therapy after speaking with them.

The proton therapy plan that was presented to me was for 44 treatments over a nine-week period, including six months of hormone therapy. Because I would need to be closer to the medical center, I decided to transfer to the Phoenix, AZ Mayo Clinic, because we have a second home in the area. It also sounded better than spending fall/winter in Rochester, MN!

The staff at both facilities was wonderful. They greeted me warmly every day, and they all knew me by name.

After my last treatment in late December 2019, my wife and I flew back home to Iowa. We celebrated a delayed Christmas with our family. I was happy to be home and it felt good to catch up with family and friends.

I'm very thankful for proton therapy, the Mayo Clinic, and support from the Brotherhood of the Balloon.

Ron Nelson
Diagnosed at age 60 in 2010
Treated at Univ. of Florida Health Proton Therapy Institute, Jacksonville, FL

"There is no way to convey in a few words how meaningful my proton therapy experience was. Suffice it to say, it changed my life."

I'm a lucky man. I'm not sure whether I feel that way in spite of having had prostate cancer, or because of it.

I was lucky to have a rare urologist who, though he was a surgeon and perfectly capable of removing my prostate, included proton therapy on the list of treatment options I should consider. At the time, I was unaware of how unusual this was. Back in 2010 when I was diagnosed, some men would only hear about proton therapy by luckily stumbling upon it during their own research.

My urologist also told me about surgery, brachytherapy, IMRT, HIFU, cryosurgery, and the possibility of active surveillance. They'd all likely work for me, he said. Spin the wheel and see where the pointer lands. He'd support my choice, and we'd take it from there.

I'm an I.T. guy, not a urologist nor an oncologist, so this decision was way outside my wheelhouse. Yet I had to decide, and ultimately, I'd have to live with my choice for the rest of my hopefully long life.

With the expectation that my Gleason 6, PSA 5.8, early diagnosed cancer could be cured, it quickly became clear that avoiding side effects was the name of the game. At merely 60 years old, everything was still working reasonably well, and I wanted to keep it that way.

I spent about a month of due diligence, researching, reading, and talking with former prostate cancer patients, as well as family and friends. Understanding that my prostate was surrounded by my bladder above, my urethra within, my rectum behind, and my nerves for sexual function around, my mission was to identify the treatment with the best shot at leaving those "organs at risk" alone.

I narrowed down my options to proton therapy and IMRT. Both were non-invasive and painless, required no anesthesia, no hospital stay, no infection risk, no injections, and no experimenting. Both had good track records of curing cancer. But unlike IMRT, proton delivered much less radiation to healthy tissue on the way to the prostate, and near zero on the way out – a major benefit. How could I not choose proton therapy?

Luckily, I live just five hours by car from one of the pioneer proton facilities: The University of Florida Health Proton Therapy Institute (UFHPTI). I made an appointment for a consultation; I was accepted as a patient; my insurance coverage was approved on the first try; and I began therapy within a few weeks. Lucky, lucky, and lucky again.

My two months at UFHPTI were incredible. Ironically, the proton therapy itself was the least eventful part of my experience. It was easy and didn't take much time out of my day. What I remember most is how I was treated on a personal level by the UFHPTI staff and the other patients. Without exception they were friendly, fun, upbeat, capable, caring, inclusive, sensitive, sincere, and available when needed for medical or personal support. Now, years later, many remain good friends.

There is no way to convey in a few words how meaningful my proton therapy experience was. Suffice it to say, it changed my life.

As a certified antisocial materialistic homebody facing an extended period away without my wife, my stuff, and my home, I expected my Jacksonville months to be lonely, isolating, and scary. It was the exact opposite. And, as a bonus it was an education in life. I learned a few things about social interaction, humility, humor, and humanity. I discovered how unimportant the material things in life are, and began to experience the joy of giving and sharing.

Because of prostate cancer and my time at UFHPTI, I've learned to appreciate life. Nearly nine years later, I've had no side effects and continue to enjoy my pre-cancer passions and pastimes— peaceful walks in the woods with my dog, Baxter, good coffee, good food, playing guitar, reading on my Kindle, and endlessly tinkering with technology. In fact, I enjoy all of this even more now, along with one new mission: the privilege of helping others in the prostate cancer world.

Most importantly, I have become a better person, even at my ripening age of 69. Acutely aware of how quickly life can change, I now enjoy every moment I have with my wife, my family, friends, and even strangers. And I am more capable of helping them to do the same.

I am a lucky man.

John Krivosheyff
Diagnosed at age 58 in 2017
Treated at Miami Cancer Institute Baptist Health South Florida in Miami, FL

"It was the best medical experience of my life."

I'm a prostate cancer survivor thanks to proton therapy and the Miami Cancer Institute. It was the best medical experience of my life.

I'm 61 and live in Fort Pierce, FL. I'm an avid golfer and travel adventurer. I retired recently and felt very lucky to have that opportunity in my early 60s. I thought my new life would be filled with birdies and pars.

But life changed when my PSA increased to a level that concerned my urologist (I'd been monitoring my PSA for 10 years). After a biopsy, it was confirmed. I had prostate cancer, Gleason score 3+3=6. I was told I could do active surveillance for a couple of years, which I accepted and began.

During that time, I started a regimen of prostate-healthy supplements like boron, Vitamin D, green tea extract EGCG, CoQ10, selenium, zinc and lycopene. I had my PSA tested every six months, and since it was decreasing, I thought the supplements were really working! But alas, two years later, my PSA went up again.

I went back to my urologist and had another biopsy, which involved 32 samples. I was told I had cancer on both sides of my prostate, and one sample was aggressive. My doctor recommended surgery. I told him I needed time to research other options.

By the grace of God, I found Bob Marckini's book, *You Can Beat Prostate Cancer,* on Amazon. My wife and I pored over the book together. By the end, we concluded that proton therapy was the only option for me.

I looked into the Miami Cancer Institute for my treatment, just 150 miles south of home. It's actually a great location for anyone as it's close to an international airport. As a bonus, while you're in treatment, you can attend Miami Heat games; do some golfing; go to the beach … and it's just a 40-minute drive to Key Largo, a dynamic tourist destination.

I met with Dr. Marcio Fagundes, radiation oncologist and proton therapy expert at MCI. He reviewed my records and answered all my

310

questions. I also met with the entire proton therapy staff. I was impressed and comforted. My wife and I knew we were in the right place.

As anticipated, my medical insurance company denied coverage for proton therapy. But the team at MCI took care of submitting an appeal, and I was relieved when my denial was overturned.

When I began my treatments, SpaceOAR gel was injected (a minor procedure to protect the rectum from radiation), as were two, tiny gold fiducials which are used to align the proton beam. A tiny dot "tattoo" was placed on each of my hips to use in alignment as well. I then had a simulation CT scan and an MRI.

My treatment started two weeks later. I was on a six-week, 28-session plan called "hypofractionation," which is shorter than the standard 44 sessions.

Overall, my proton therapy experience was seamless (only once was my bladder overfilled). Each treatment lasted about a half hour, and then I was able to hit golf balls or visit the gym (I joined one for the month). Surprisingly, the time went by quickly.

I can't accurately describe the level of competence and caring displayed by every member of my treatment staff – the doctors, medical assistants, nurses and radiation technicians were incredible. Their healing, loving hands guided me every step of the way through my proton treatment. I highly recommend the Miami Cancer Institute.

Brent Holsten
Diagnosed at age 47 in 2019
Treated at the Emory Proton Center, Atlanta, GA

"Do your due diligence. Learn about all the treatment options so you can find the one that's best for you. Then choose the treatment that'll help you sleep at night. I did – and it was proton therapy."

Bob Marckini's first edition of *You Can Beat Prostate Cancer* changed my life. And later, so did proton therapy. So, when I was asked to write a testimonial for the second edition about my experiences with prostate cancer and proton therapy, I jumped at the chance.

I am one of the younger prostate cancer patients. I was diagnosed when I was 47. I had a PSA of 3.9 and a Gleason score of 3+3=6. I'm a third-generation prostate cancer patient.

Like many, I thought I knew what was best – surgery. And I'd planned on it because I'd watched my father fight prostate cancer for 14 years. I knew my time would probably come. And my father, along with everyone else I knew, had undergone surgery. It's also what my urologist recommended.

When a friend sent me Bob's book, I realized there were other options to consider. They all seemed to have similar cure rates, but the side effects were different. Proton stuck out as the procedure with the least number of side effects for the short- and long-term. So, I took Bob Marckini's advice and spoke with former patients. I also kept other treatments on the table to make sure I was really choosing the best option for me. I met with various doctors specializing in each.

No matter what I read or who I talked to, I kept going back to proton therapy because I was convinced that side effects would be minimal, if at all. Eventually, I selected the Emory Proton Treatment Center in Atlanta, GA. I had an uncle and cousins who lived nearby, and I found that comforting. Also, from the very beginning, every single person I met at Emory seemed to really care about me – I wasn't just a "number."

It was decided that, because my cancer stage was low, I'd undergo the shorter hypofractionated treatment protocol rather than the standard 44 sessions. My program would include just 28 treatments.

Once I decided on Emory, the first step was getting my health insurance to pay for the procedure. Emory had two amazing women whose job was to deal with the insurance companies. They said it could take up to 14 days to get approval, they did it nine. Once approved, I had to get SpaceOAR gel (to protect my rectum from radiation), and they put three carbon markers in my prostate. It was a 15-minute procedure. If you go through this, bring headphones and music to listen to – you'll want to be distracted. A few days later, I had a CT scan and MRI simulation. Fourteen days later, I was ready to start my treatments.

Once I arrived in Atlanta, I'd start each day swimming with a local masters group. Then I'd head over to Emory. If I had time, I'd get a coffee and head downstairs to the men's lounge – a room with seating and a TV. You always knew the prostate patients, because we all had to wear two robes and just socks.

From the time I walked into the room for treatment until the time I walked out, I listened to about two songs on my headphones; That's about seven minutes.

Once a week, I'd play golf. With the combination of the swimming, the commuting, and my daily treatments, I was tired by the end of the day. For me, stairs were my nemesis. I never avoided them; I just knew I'd be short of breath when I reached the top. As the days and weeks passed, my strength and stamina returned.

Emory worked for me. I couldn't be happier with the choice I made. With the shorter treatment cycle and the southern hospitality, I was smiling most of the time. I wrote a blog about my experience. You can find it here: https://prostatecancerat47.blogspot.com/

I want to reiterate that none of this would have happened if I hadn't read Bob Marckini's first edition of *You Can Beat Prostate Cancer*. It reminds me of the old saying: "The more you know, the more you realize you don't know." Do your due diligence. Learn about all the treatment options so you can find the one that's best for you. Then choose the treatment that'll help you sleep at night. I did – and it was proton therapy.

Bob Reimer
Diagnosed at age 67 in 1998
Treated at Loma Linda Univ. Cancer Center, Loma Linda, CA

PSA 61: *"You have Gleason 10 prostate cancer and have one to three years to live. . . That was 21 years ago."*

My urologist started the conversation with, "You have Gleason 10 prostate cancer and have one to three years to live. Go home and get your affairs in order." That was 21 years ago.

I had physicals every year, but was never told my PSA. I worried about prostate cancer and asked my doctor repeatedly if I should be screened. His answer was always, "Your prostate is slightly enlarged, but normal for your age." I was 66.

In December 1997, my internist thought I may have an infection because my PSA had spiked more so than usual – *it was 61.* I started 10 days of antibiotics. Upon having a re-test shortly thereafter, my doctor told me to see a urologist ASAP.

In January, I had a biopsy. I met with my urologist to review the results. He said, "You have Gleason 10 prostate cancer and have one to three years to live. Go home and get your affairs in order."

My wife Audrey and I were *shocked.* After all, I *felt good* and had *no symptoms.*

I immediately started on the hormone, Zolodex, and started researching treatment options.

I had a friend who'd gone to Loma Linda University Cancer Center for proton treatment a year earlier. He told me he'd had a great experience and was cancer-free, so I made an appointment for a consultation. I spent an hour with the doctor. He answered all my questions and was very honest with me; Since my cancer was so aggressive, he felt I probably wouldn't be a candidate for proton treatment since the cancer was most likely *outside my prostate.* However, he ordered a "prostascint" scan of my entire torso to make sure. Much to my surprise (and joy), the results showed the cancer was *still localized. Audrey and I were thrilled.*

I started proton therapy early July 1998. The only side effects I experienced were diarrhea that lasted a short time. Since treatment, my PSA has gone down continually, and I've had no further side effects.

Audrey and I felt God's presence guiding us through this time in our lives. The prayers and support of friends and family, and the wonderful care and love shown to us at LLUCC have been beyond description. God is good.

I'm 88 now, and it's been 21 years since my treatment. I'm still a huge supporter of proton therapy, Loma Linda, and T*he Brotherhood of the Balloon.* For years, I've volunteered to speak with newly diagnosed men, answer their questions, and set their minds at ease. I'm in touch with Bob Marckini and Deb Hickey at the BOB often – sometimes just to say hello. Although I've slowed down a bit, I'm still active in my community and able to take care of my lovely wife, who's been ill.

Ron Hammer
Diagnosed at age 60 in 2011
Treated at MD Anderson, Houston, TX

"I can't imagine a better treatment option than proton therapy."

I was diagnosed with prostate cancer in 2011 – Gleason 3+3=6. As an engineer, I'd done a lot of research on treatment options, including reading Bob Marckini's book, *You Can Beat Prostate Cancer.* My findings led me to proton therapy and MD Anderson in Houston.

To my surprise, the doctor at MDA suggested I consider Active Surveillance since my disease was low-grade. He then offered, if my disease progressed, I may be a candidate for a clinical trial investigating the effectiveness of hypofractionated proton therapy. This shortened-treatment protocol reduced the number of sessions from 44 (standard of care) down to just 15, at twice the dosage, administered every other day for about five weeks. This sounded good to me since I was still employed and could work remotely from my apartment.

I stayed on Active Surveillance for three years and saw my local urologist to administer the required annual biopsies. Results from my last biopsy with him indicated that the disease had progressed to an intermediate-risk level of Gleason 7 (4+3). It was time to pull the trigger and return to MDA.

But, nothing's ever easy. I had a couple of other problems. My prostate was too large for effective proton therapy and had to be reduced in size. In order to do this, I received one dose of Lupron and waited another three months for it to do its job. To make matters worse, I was notified that my insurance (United Healthcare) wouldn't cover proton therapy. Fortunately, MDA has a dedicated team of people who files insurance appeals on behalf of patients at no additional charge. I felt confident that they'd help me obtain coverage.

At the end of the three months on Lupron, and after the third appeal, I was notified that UHC would cover the clinical trial. They also covered my airfare between Kansas City and Houston, as well as my apartment rental in Houston.

When the Lupron had done its job and my prostate gland was reduced to 40cc, I began proton therapy in April 2015. I came home six weeks later.

My experience at MDA was nothing short of amazing. Everything ran like clockwork. The entire medical staff was kind and knowledgeable. The most amazing part was the camaraderie among the men in my treatment group. We listened to each other's personal stories, and told a ton of jokes. On one occasion, we were laughing so wildly, a nurse asked us to tone it down because patients down the hall thought we were having a party.

My PSA dropped from 5.88 prior to treatment down to just under 1.0, where it remains. I can't imagine a better treatment option than proton therapy.

Charles Stohrer
Diagnosed at age 45 in 2014
Treated at Loma Linda Univ. Cancer Center, Loma Linda, CA

"Diagnosed at 45—I was shocked!"

When I was diagnosed with prostate cancer on Feb. 9, 2014, I was shocked! I didn't have any symptoms; I was in great shape; and suddenly, there was this blood test that said I had cancer. I didn't know what to think. I was just 45, a senior design manager, and an active athlete.

I was in the prime of my life!

My urologist encouraged me to have surgery. I figured he knew best, so I scheduled the operation.

I realized later that newly diagnosed men need to consider the *side effects* of the treatment options. Each modality seems to have similar cure rates – *but what about the side effects?* My advice is to ask your urologist: "If you had prostate cancer, what would *you* do?" Make sure he looks you in the eye when he answers.

After scheduling my surgery, I sent an email to several friends, telling them about my diagnosis and asking them to pray for me. All were encouraging, but two of them were especially supportive. The first was my girlfriend, Laura. She told me we'd get through this together. Ironically, Laura's father was diagnosed with prostate cancer two weeks later. The two of us suddenly had a lot to talk about. The second was a friend of mine. His father had gone to Loma Linda University Cancer Center for proton therapy *14 years ago* and he was doing great. He sent me a link to their website and suggested I watch some of their video testimonials. Three days later, I bought a plane ticket to California (from Kalamazoo, MI). After my consult, I canceled my surgery appointment.

During my proton treatment, *everyone* was helpful. LLUCC's "Make Man Whole" mission is extraordinary. In order to make patients feel at home, they arrange group activities including restaurant tours, mountain hikes and support group meetings. They also offer programs on diet and lifestyle. All of this creates a spirit of camaraderie and esprit de corps. Even though I didn't know anyone in Loma Linda prior to my treatment, I never once felt isolated or lonely.

I worked out every day during my treatment at LLUCC's Drayson Fitness Center (free for patients). I also worked full-time (remotely). In between taking advantage of the gym facility, all the activities and working, I also enjoyed time with my girlfriend. She flew out to meet me for 10 days during the sixth week of my 10-week treatment program.

Two days after my treatment ended on May 14, I turned 46. Four months after that, my doctor ordered a PSA test. I was hoping my PSA had dropped 30 to 50 percent. But it was even better than that!

Today, I feel great and I've had no side effects. I ate well before treatment, but I eat better now. I was in shape before treatment, but I'm in better shape now. Life is good! If I'm not at the gym, I'm with my beautiful girlfriend and a great group of friends. We go to the beach and go boating in the summer. In the winter, I snow board. We also take plenty of vacations. For my 50th birthday, Laura surprised me with a trip to Tahiti!

I volunteer as a reference on LLUCC's and the BOB's former proton patient reference list. I also volunteer with the Imerman Angels One-on-One Cancer Support Group. A lot of guys come to me in their mid-40s and early 50s. I enjoy helping them find their way to proton therapy.

Here's my advice to every man: Have your PSA checked and monitored as early as 40 – especially if you have prostate cancer in your family. Then, you can establish a base line to follow. Hopefully, your PSA will never change. Luckily, my doctor checked mine at 43. If I had waited until 50, I believe I'd have a very different story to tell, if any at all.

Douglas A. Palecek
Diagnosed at age 62 in 2012
Treated at the Northwestern Med. Proton Center, Chicago, IL

"Would I make the same treatment decision again? Without a doubt. I have friends who've had surgery and others who've had IMRT; None of them are happy with their choice."

I was diagnosed with prostate cancer in early 2012. My PSA was 6.4; my Gleason score was 8, and I was a T2b/c. The doctor recommended surgery or IMRT, but I was unsure, so I did my own research and found proton therapy. I chose the treatment due to the accuracy of the beam and the prospect of little-to-no side effects.

I was treated with proton therapy at the Northwestern Medicine Proton Center in March 2012. Treatment was a breeze. I had mild side effects – urinary/bowel urgency right after treatment – which went away quickly with a simple drug treatment.

For the past seven years since my proton treatment, I've had no further side effects and my PSA is 0.137.

Would I make the same treatment decision again? Without a doubt. I have friends who've had surgery and others who've had IMRT; none of them are happy with their choice.

Hopefully, my testimonial will encourage others to do their own homework, read Bob's book, and consider proton therapy.

Steve Peterson
Diagnosed at age 65 in 2017
Treated at Penn Medicine Roberts Proton Therapy Center in Philadelphia, PA

"My best advice: There can be only one advocate for decisions about your health and that is you. Educate yourself. Find the best solution for you. I believe I did that in selecting proton therapy."

I was diagnosed with prostate cancer in 2016, with a Gleason score of 6 and a PSA that never exceeded 3.75. A subsequent MRI and biopsy in early 2017 resulted in a Gleason score of 8. Clinically I was diagnosed as T1C.

My urologist suggested surgery for those under 65 and conventional radiation for those over 65. Fortunately, I'd started my homework immediately and had read Bob Marckini's book. Incidentally, I was already convinced that proton therapy was the right approach regardless of my age. I was 65; Medicare would cover it; And I was a 45-minute train ride from Penn Medicine's Roberts Proton Therapy Center.

I met with an oncologist at Penn in February 2017. He examined all my test results, MRIs, and biopsies, and determined I was a Gleason 7, not 8. I sent my slides to Johns Hopkins for a third and final confirmation on my Gleason score and they confirmed Gleason 7. I highly recommend sending your biopsy slides to Johns Hopkins for a second opinion no matter what your Gleason score is! Although the proton therapy plan wouldn't change between Gleason 7 and 8, the duration of hormone treatments prescribed was only three months. If I was a Gleason 8, I would have been on hormones for 12 months.

Treatment was easy and the 44 days went by more quickly than I expected. My treatment times varied from evening to afternoons to mornings, and I met all the technicians over the nine weeks I was there. They were all wonderful people and made my experience as enjoyable as it could be.

On a side note, I can't write this testimonial without mentioning the wonderful patients, especially the children, I met during my treatment at Penn. These people were there under the most serious conditions, with proton therapy being a key treatment for their survival. Spending time with them and their loved ones was a sobering experience and made my condition seem a lesser concern compared to the challenges many of them faced. Everyone was so hopeful for what proton therapy could do for them. I'll never forget that experience.

After treatment, my PSA bounced slightly from 0.1 to 0.7 the first year, but dropped the second year. My most recent PSA was indetectable at <0.1. I've had no side effects, which was my main reason for selecting proton therapy versus traditional photon radiation.

A final word: my brother-in-law had a radical prostatectomy four years ago. He was a Gleason 7 as well. He was 60 years old, still working, not on Medicare, and his medical insurance wouldn't cover proton therapy. He's the person who sent me Bob Marckini's book. I think that saved my life. Sadly, he's had a recurrence and is evaluating treatments again. It's my hope that he can have proton therapy for salvage treatment.

My best advice: There can be only *one advocate* for decisions about your health and that is you. Educate yourself. Find the best solution for you. I believe I did that in selecting proton therapy.

Jim Haigh
Diagnosed at age 71 in 2014
Treated at the Oklahoma Proton Center, Oklahoma City, OK

"… I'm a strong proponent of proton therapy. I had absolutely no side effects at all."

I flew in South Vietnam in 1965-66 and was exposed to Agent Orange. There's some speculation that this chemical agent could be a contributor to prostate cancer.

I was diagnosed with prostate cancer in early 2014. My Gleason score was 7. My PSA was 1.6 in 2008, but gradually increased to 4.3 by the time of my diagnosis. My local oncologist wanted to do surgery. When I learned I'd most likely need blood after the procedure, I decided that wasn't the best option for me.

I then visited with a friend from Oklahoma City who'd undergone surgery to remove his prostate. He was not pleased with the results. He introduced me to the Oklahoma Proton Center. While considering proton treatment, I picked up a copy of Bob Marckini's book, *You Can Beat Prostate Cancer.* That was all I needed to make my final determination – I was going to have proton therapy. I'd like to add that Bob's book is a must-read for anyone facing prostate cancer.

I traveled back and forth from my hometown of Springfield, MO, to Oklahoma for treatments. The folks at the proton center were kind enough to work with me to schedule my appointments according to my commute.

The Oklahoma Proton Center is super nice; It's well maintained, and the staff is great. It was a good experience for me, and I'd recommend the facility to others interested in proton therapy.

I had 44 treatments. My latest PSA is 0.2. Now age 76, I'm a strong proponent of proton therapy. I had absolutely no side effects at all.

Bruce D. Schrimpf
Diagnosed at age 72 in 2018
Treated at the Mayo Clinic in Rochester, MN

"Since I'd had precision proton beam radiation already, it was possible to undergo that same effective treatment again without concern about repeat radiation."

I had proton therapy twice.

In the summer of 2017, my voice suddenly sounded like I had a bad case of laryngitis. I couldn't speak normally – I sounded a bit like Mickey Mouse. I knew something was very wrong. And since I'm a lawyer, I speak in public for a living, so my situation was even more concerning.

I went to a major teaching hospital in Milwaukee, WI, and was told I had a paraganglioma that was growing on my right vagus nerve. I was told surgery was out of the question and that my best option was radiation therapy. I was given a referral to the Mayo Clinic in Rochester, MN.

In September, I met with a doctor at the Mayo Clinic. He suggested I consider proton beam therapy. Because my rare, benign tumor developed close to crucial nerves and tissues, including my salivary glands, proton therapy could be effective and well-tolerated because of its pinpoint accuracy.

I began proton therapy in October 2017, and completed my treatments in early December, a total of 27 sessions with three administrations of the beam each time. I have had no side effects from the treatment; My salivary glands were spared because of the precision of the beam. My voice, while somewhat different, and with the help of adjunct physical therapy, was back.

Recently, I spoke twice to a group of military reservists about legal rights under the Uniformed Services Employment and Reemployment Rights Act. The rooms had no microphones and I had to present to 100-plus personnel. I did fine.

A very smart neurologist at the Mayo Clinic was concerned that I may have more paragangliomas, and ordered a full body PET Scan. Two suspicious areas were found – one on my lung that turned out to be an infection (later treated with antibiotics), and another that turned out to be prostate cancer. I was a Gleason 5+4=9, T2C, with prostatic extension and possible lymph node involvement. My PSA was 12.3.

Since I'd had precision proton beam radiation already, it was possible to undergo that same effective treatment again without concern about repeat radiation. I started Lupron on Dec. 5, 2017, and commenced 26 sessions of proton therapy on Jan. 28, 2018.

My latest PSA was 0.1, and I plan to get checked every three months. I'm hopeful this therapy has done its magic twice.

Rees Harward
Diagnosed at age 66 in 2016
Treated at the Texas Center for Proton Therapy, Irving, TX

"It still bothers me that some doctors suggest treatments simply because it's the treatment they specialize in, and not what might be best for their patients. You must be your own advocate. I'm fortunate to have learned that early on."

I was diagnosed with prostate cancer on March 8, 2016. My PSA was 8.6 with 10 of 12 biopsy cores positive. Four cores scored 4+3. I held this information from everyone except immediate family. My wife and I didn't know what to make of my diagnosis and had no idea what we were going to do about it. I remember feeling scared, apprehensive, and somewhat in denial.

My urologist told me that surgery was my best option. Fortunately, there were two life experiences I'd had that prompted me to question his suggestion.

My father, who passed in 1998, was a family physician in southern California. You'd think I'd believe a doctor's opinion is gospel having had a father who was a doctor. But I remember my dad making house calls in the '50s and '60s. When he knew he couldn't help a patient, he'd recognize his limits and send them to a major hospital, like Loma Linda University Health, where they could get the care they needed. This told me his patients and their needs were his priority; He didn't always assume he knew best.

The other experience I had was with my youngest son. He was born with a serious heart defect. His doctor told us he had to have surgery immediately or he'd die. Then he said something that might be surprising to some, but not to me because I'd grown up watching my father, who would have said the same thing.

My son's doctor suggested my son not be treated at the hospital where he worked because they didn't have much experience with the surgical procedure my son needed. Instead, the doctor recommended a hospital in Birmingham, AL. The pediatric cardiologist there was the one who developed the surgical procedure, and he knew it would be the best care for my son.

We were on a plane that afternoon. Thirty years later, my son is healthy and living a normal life, thanks to that doctor who cared more about his patient than the hospital he worked for.

Back to my prostate cancer: I remember my urologist tiptoeing around the various treatment options and then strongly recommending surgery (because that's what his group did).

Later that day, I began my own research on surgery. I also looked at other treatment options. I met with three surgeons and a radiation specialist, but I still wasn't convinced on which treatment to choose, so I continued my hunt online.

I also made it my mission to speak with as many former patients, representing each treatment option I was considering, as I could find. Note I asked one of the surgeons to speak with his former patients and was told he couldn't offer that to me. I scratched that practice off my list as I walked out of his office.

The men I spoke with were extremely helpful in my decision-making process.

I found proton therapy and the Loma Linda University Cancer Center website during an Internet search one day. I remembered immediately that Loma Linda was the hospital my father would send his patients to and a lightbulb went on. After digging a little further, I found the ProtonBob.com website, which led me to the Texas Center for Proton Therapy – just a half hour from my home in Midlothian. Everything was coming together. It didn't take me long to call and make an appointment.

I began my treatment program – a combination of hormonal therapy and proton therapy – in May 2017. I drove 35 miles to and from the Texas Center for Proton Therapy from my home, Monday through Friday, for my 15 – 20-minute treatments. There were absolutely no restrictions; I had minimal side effects; and I continued to work and play golf.

Today I had my three-year exam. My PSA is 0.46 and I couldn't be happier. Other than mild proctitis, which has cleared up, I've had no long-term side effects.

It still bothers me that some doctors suggest treatments simply because it's the treatment they specialize in, and not what might be best for their patients. You must be your own advocate. I'm fortunate to have learned that early on.

My experience with prostate cancer and my treatment at Texas Center for Proton Therapy has made my wife and me stronger in our faith. We're so thankful to have witnessed God's hand at work at the Texas Center, especially with the children. In fact, I've thought many times that God allowed proton therapy to be developed for children. I, and a lot of other old farts, are just a side benefit of proton therapy.

Bruce Hill
Diagnosed at age 69 in 2017
Treated at the Maryland Proton Treatment Center, Baltimore, MD

"My advice for anyone with a prostate cancer diagnosis. Never give up – keep fighting! And consider proton beam radiation therapy!"

I'm an attorney in Baltimore City, MD. When I was diagnosed with prostate cancer, I wanted a non-surgical (non-invasive) treatment option that would allow me to keep my commitment to my clients.

Online research led me to two books written by prostate cancer survivors: Ron Nelson's *Protons vs. Prostate Cancer: EXPOSED* and Robert Marckini's *You Can Beat Prostate Cancer: And You Don't Need Surgery to Do It*. Both men had received proton therapy. I was interested in the treatment because it could target my prostate cancer while minimizing damage to healthy surrounding tissues, thereby reducing the risks for side effects.

I learned there was a proton facility in my home state – the Maryland Proton Treatment Center. I found their website, filled out a consultation request, and booked an appointment. Within a few hours, a nurse called to learn more about my diagnosis. She recommended I come in for a consultation.

After that meeting, I'd made my decision and became a patient in May 2017. I'd go in every morning at 7:20 a.m. for my treatment. By 8:00 a.m. I was on my way to work. I tolerated the treatments well. In fact, other than getting up a bit earlier than usual, my schedule was quite routine.

I have nothing but praise for proton therapy and the Maryland Proton Treatment Center. I've never been to a medical facility where everyone is so caring, kind and compassionate. It was like the TV show, *Cheers.* Everybody knew my name – the valet guy, the front desk staff, the nurses – they all said, "Good morning, Mr. Hill" when I arrived.

My treatment ended in July 2017. Since then, I've retired and moved to Delaware. I spend my time riding my bicycle and my motorcycle and enjoying the beach near my home.

My advice for anyone with a prostate cancer diagnosis. Never give up – keep fighting! And consider proton beam radiation therapy!

Walt Wagner
Diagnosed at age 67 in 2014
Treated at California Protons, San Diego, CA

Walt had proton salvage treatment following robotic surgery for prostate cancer.

I spent much of my life as a quintessential adult male, doing stupid stuff that wears out some of the moving parts of this incredible body we're blessed with. I had no major health issues (until prostate cancer) – I blew out my knee skiing and later wiped out the last bit of cartilage in my hip on the tennis court. After a couple years of suffering, hoping my hip would improve with physical therapy, I finally went to an orthopedic surgeon who suggested a hip replacement. In preparing for the surgery, I made a long overdue appointment with my family doctor. He ran some simple tests (that I should've done much earlier).

Sure enough, the blood test indicated that my PSA was in the mid-teens, so my doctor referred me to a urologist who conducted only the second DRE I'd ever had (the previous one was decades earlier). The DRE indicated an abnormality, so the next step was a biopsy. Cancer was present in my prostate with a Gleason score of 7.

Since I was familiar with the Scripps health network in San Diego, I decided to consult with them on the various options for treatment. At the time, the Scripps Proton Therapy Center (now California Protons) hadn't been completed, so my choices were limited to more traditional treatments. I elected to have my prostate removed with a robotic prostatectomy.

The surgery went okay, though I had some undesirable side effects. My PSA fell to below 0.1, but then started to climb. Shortly thereafter, my urologic oncology surgeon told me the surgery hadn't removed all the cancer (I learned later that statistically, 70 percent of the time errant cells remain in the prostate bed after surgery). He referred me to Dr. Carl Rossi at CA Protons. Dr. Rossi proposed a series of 36 proton therapy treatments to blanket that area.

The doctors and staff at CA Protons were simply amazing. They offered tours of the facility and gave presentations on the science involved in proton therapy. I met with the entire staff that would be involved in my treatment including the physicists. Over the course of my treatment, the technicians that worked with me daily were professional and caring.

I was thrilled to ring the bell on the last day of my treatments in February 2015. It was just days before my daughter's wedding on Valentine's Day. I continued to follow up with Dr. Rossi for several months as my PSA dropped to undetectable levels.

Thank you, proton therapy, Dr. Rossi and your incredible staff at CA Protons. I now live a very active life – playing tennis, hiking, dancing, and traveling

Charles F. DeMailly Jr.
Diagnosed at age 59 in 2002
Treated at Massachusetts General Hospital, Boston, MA

"I am a living example of the fact that it works, and it certainly preserves the quality of your life."

328

A routine blood test showed a 3.9 PSA. My urologist prescribed a biopsy, which confirmed prostate cancer. My urologist recommended surgery, just as my good friend, Bob Marckini, said he would. Bob gave me a copy of his book, and after reading it, I was convinced proton therapy was the best option for me. But, living in Massachusetts, I was faced with a dilemma.

I had recently purchased a small business; I was working over 100 hours a week and needed to stay close to home to run the business. So, Loma Linda in Southern California was out of the question.

The only other proton center in the country, Massachusetts General Hospital in Boston, had recently opened and was within driving distance of my home. So, the choice was easy.

Bob put me in touch with Dr. Anthony Zietman at Mass. General and things moved quickly. I soon began my treatment with a 7:00 am start time. This worked well, because it allowed me to be at work by 8:30 am. Toward the end of my eight weeks of treatment I experienced some slight fatigue, but I never missed a day of work and things at my business ran smoothly.

Proton therapy is quick and painless. Side effects were minimal – urinary urgency was a temporary issue, but over time became a non-issue.

Dr. Zietman and the people at Mass. General were wonderful. I highly recommend proton therapy for prostate cancer and am a living example of the fact that it works, and it certainly preserves the quality of your life.

James Bodino
Diagnosed at age 70 in 2012
Treated at ProCure Proton Therapy Center, New Jersey

"At the time of my diagnosis, I never thought, nearly eight years later, I'd be a healthy man with a PSA reading of 0.05."

I was diagnosed with high-risk prostate cancer in May 2012 at the age of 70. To say I was shocked and feared for my life would be a gross understatement. Since my cancer was so advanced, the treatment options presented to me were surgical removal or conventional radiation. I was not offered proton radiation because I was told it was "in the embryonic stage."

Fortunately, my daughter was the office manager for two radiologists in New Jersey. They both recommended I investigate the ProCure Proton Therapy Center in Somerset.

Within a few days I met with the director of the center. He immediately alleviated my fears. A PowerPoint presentation he showed me answered my unasked questions and more. After the consultation, I was convinced proton radiation would be my best option and I scheduled my treatments.

On my first day of treatment, I remember feeling much trepidation. Fortunately, my brother lived only a half hour from the treatment center, which gave me comfort and made daily travel easy. Also, my wife was there to lend her support. We were pleasantly surprised by the reception we received when we entered the lobby that day. The office manager and staff welcomed us with warm smiles and words of encouragement. Their goodwill made the process easier on both of us.

The technicians were part of what I refer to as my "ProCure family." They were not only efficient; They were compassionate. They offered to play music during my treatments, thoughtfully selecting songs from the '50s. However, I insisted they play music they listen to – today's top hits. Ever since, I've become a big fan of Adele.

At my first treatment, I also remember the technician holding a 12-inch tube – the balloon. I think she noticed my eyes bulge, because she carefully explained how and why it's used. The balloon is inserted in the rectum and filled with air. The purpose is to protect the rectum to allow the beam to pinpoint the tumor without collateral damage. Painful? No. Unpleasant? Somewhat.

The side effects during and shortly after the treatments were minimal, but since I'd undergone hormonal therapy, I had some hot flashes. I now appreciate what women endure during menopause. I also experienced some dysfunctional erection shortly after treatment, but like the hot flashes, that subsided in time. During treatment, I golfed, swam and walked.

I strongly believe without receiving proton therapy I wouldn't be alive. At the time of my diagnosis, I never thought, nearly eight years later, I'd be a healthy man with a PSA reading of 0.05. I'm thankful for proton therapy and the ProCure Proton Therapy Center.

Bob Richburg
Diagnosed at age 72 in 2017
Treated at Ackerman Cancer Center in Jacksonville, FL

"I didn't suffer from any side effects, which allowed me to enjoy daily walks. My wife and I spent our days in Jacksonville as if we were on vacation."

My wife and I spent the summer of 2017 in Jacksonville, FL, so I could be treated for prostate cancer with proton therapy at the Ackerman Cancer Center. I learned about proton therapy years earlier after a friend was successfully treated at Loma Linda University Cancer Center in California.

When I was diagnosed at age 72, I immediately began researching proton therapy in my home state of Florida. I discovered, and became fascinated with, Ackerman because it was a privately owned facility, the only one of its kind in the U.S. I left a telephone message on a Sunday, expecting a response the following week. My wife and I were delighted when we heard back from someone that afternoon! Within a week, we drove four and a half hours to Jacksonville for a consultation.

From the greeting we received from the receptionists to our first meeting with Dr. Scot Ackerman, my wife and I were impressed. Everyone was friendly, supportive, respectful, and caring. The atmosphere was comforting, and it soon became clear that this is where I wanted to be treated.

Friends lent us a condo nearby and within 20 days, we returned to Jacksonville for my treatment. I was one of the first Ackerman patients to receive the SpaceOAR hydrogel option that provides space between the rectum and the prostate, making it much less likely that the rectum is exposed to radiation.

I received 45 treatments. During my time at Ackerman, I grew to know and appreciate the technicians and other health professionals who took care of me. I didn't suffer from any side effects, which allowed me to enjoy daily walks. My wife and I spent our days in Jacksonville as if we were on vacation.

Since my treatment, I continue to work with my mediation business and play on my hobby farm. I wholeheartedly recommend proton therapy at the Ackerman Cancer Center – it's a gem!

Allan J. Kuipers
Diagnosed at age 67 in 2014
Treated at Seattle Cancer Care Alliance Proton Therapy Center, Seattle, WA

"It's important to note that proton therapy just became part of my daily routine; I'd stop on the way home from work. The average treatment time took about 15 minutes."

After a routine physical, I was diagnosed with prostate cancer on Oct. 31, 2014. My Gleason score was 7 (4+3) and my PSA was 5.95. In reflection, it seems appropriate that I got the scare of my life on Halloween.

I spent the rest of the year evaluating treatment options. My urologist gave me the names of two doctors – one specialized in radiation (photon) and the other in brachytherapy. I quickly ruled out photon radiation because of the potential damage to healthy tissues. Then I learned the radioactive seeds (brachytherapy) could migrate to other parts of the body (I read somewhere that they burned through someone's bladder), so I ruled that out too.

I kept researching and found two more options – da Vinci laparoscopic surgery and proton therapy. Then I read some more patient horror stories relating to surgery and focused on proton therapy because it appeared to be minimally invasive, if at all, and had the least potential for side effects. It was pin-point treatment that attacked the bad tissue without damaging the good.

In January 2015, I began six months of hormone therapy to suppress testosterone, a breeding ground for cancer. Two months later, I began 44 days of proton treatments, finishing on May 15. It's important to note that proton therapy just became part of my daily routine; I'd stop on the way home from work. The average treatment time took about 15 minutes.

My side effects were minimal – a bit of urinary frequency and slight burning. Flomax was helpful. I also had a few hot flashes as the result of the hormonal therapy. That dissipated a few months after I had my last shot.

I feel blessed to have had proton therapy. If I were diagnosed tomorrow, I'd choose the same treatment. My latest PSA was 0.2. I'm a cancer survivor!

I owe my life to the wonderful doctors, nurses and radiation therapists at the Seattle proton center.

John Miller
Diagnosed at age 70 in 2017
Treated at University Hospital Seidman Cancer Center in Cleveland, OH

"So, the testimonials I read about proton therapy proved to be true in my experience."

When I was age 68 (2014), I began proactively researching prostate cancer treatment options as my PSA was rising. A few years later, a biopsy confirmed my fears. However, I was still confused about the myriad treatment options because virtually all of them produced side effects I didn't want to live with. The only option that seemed reasonable was proton therapy. I'd read Bob Marckini's book, *You*

Can Beat Prostate Cancer, and spoke with a former proton patient from Arizona. Their experiences matched.

Still, I wanted to cover all my bases, so I met with a conventional radiation oncologist. He just solidified my opinion of their approach, which included their polite but obvious disdain for anything outside their services. When I brought up proton therapy, he said it was "too new, too unproven, too undocumented, too expensive, and too remotely available." But I was still interested in proton and willing to travel anywhere and undergo three months of treatment if it meant my quality of life would be maintained. As luck would have it, I didn't have to travel outside of Ohio where I lived. Upon further investigation, I found a proton therapy center in Cleveland.

A phone call got me an appointment within the week. Three weeks later, I began my proton treatment at University Hospital Seidman Cancer Center in October 2017. Nine weeks went by amazingly fast. The staff was exceptional in helping me to obtain medical insurance coverage and coordinating my treatment schedules. I might add: considering the unpredictable Ohio winter weather, the staff was wonderfully accommodating in meeting my travel needs as I had a 320-mile daily commute.

So, the testimonials I read about proton therapy proved to be true in my experience. Treatments were handled quickly, never exceeding 30 minutes, and I had absolutely zero side effects or any associated discomfort. Plus, my dear wife got to shop every trip and I got to enjoy a different cuisine just as often.

Today I've got nothing but good news to report: no limitations, no side effects, and a scheduled multi-destination 50th wedding anniversary cruising celebration coming up. What could possibly be better than that?

James Meares, DDS
Diagnosed at age 73 in 2013
Treated at Hampton University Proton Therapy Institute, Hampton, VA

"I can't stress enough the benefits of proton therapy – it's effective, non-traumatic and has minimal, if any, side effects. I've had patients and friends who've regretted not having proton therapy; They chose other modalities and are all suffering from side effects."

I was diagnosed with two different types of cancer in 2013. The first was mantle cell lymphoma and the second, prostate cancer. Both appeared to be the result of serving in Viet Nam as a Naval Officer serving on a destroyer in the mid-60s. The ship anchored in Da Nang harbor several times, and although the water that we drank was distilled on board the ship, the Agent Orange wasn't broken down or removed, and thus the entire crew was exposed to the chemical agent.

At the time of my diagnosis, I was in practice as a general and cosmetic dentist in Virginia Beach, VA.

After receiving the news of my dual malignancies, I began to search for oncologists, hematologists, and urologists to determine how I should confront these challenges. It was suggested I have the mantle cell lymphoma treated with chemotherapy first, and then investigate prostate cancer treatment options. My urologist suggested robotic surgery, traditional radiation therapy, or brachytherapy, but I wasn't sold on any of them.

Prior to attending dental school, I'd earned an MS in immunology. I knew that after chemotherapy with Ibrutinib and Bendamustine, my immune system would be compromised. Any invasive approach, such as prostatectomy or placing seeds in the prostate gland, would carry the potential for infection. Adding radiation therapy would also create an environment for post-treatment infection. In fact, I'd experienced a severe prostate infection after a biopsy soon after the completion of chemotherapy. I was treated with IV antibiotics through a port. It took six weeks to heal and I was bed ridden.

While at home recovering, I searched for alternative prostate cancer treatment options and stumbled upon the Protonbob.com website. I read about proton therapy and learned the delivery was precise, non-invasive, and the potential for side effects was minimal. This was important because my lymphoma could only be controlled, not cured. Proton therapy gave me hope.

Fortunately, my urologist was aware of the Hampton University Proton Therapy Institute (HUPTI) in Hampton, VA. Although he thought the treatment was novel, he referred me to a radiation oncologist at the facility and I was on my way.

My experience at HUPTI was world class. My team of radiation oncologists, technicians, nurses, and even the engineers was outstanding. They were compassionate and explained the treatment with clarity and professionalism. In this day of advanced technology, my treatment approach was high tech and high touch – the treatment was efficient and effective.

I had my daily treatments in the middle of the day, which allowed me to see my dental patients in the morning. Most importantly, I didn't experience any side effects and was able to carry on with my regular activities.

Since treatment, my PSA dropped continually. Today, there is no evidence of prostate cancer. I can't stress enough the benefits of proton therapy – it's effective, non-traumatic and has minimal, if any, side effects. I've had patients and friends who've regretted not having proton therapy; They chose other modalities and are all suffering from side effects.

I am blessed to have a supportive wife and family. I transitioned out of my practice about five years ago and I'm enjoying retirement. My wife and I are involved in our church choir; We travel often to visit relatives in Greece; And we spend a lot of time with our two grandsons. I'm an avid reader of history and science fiction and enjoy daily walks and going to the gym. At age 79, I feel great. Although I still have future challenges with the lymphoma, I'm hopeful that I'll continue the path that I'm on.

Visit www.protonbob.com/testimonials
to read 130 additional testimonials

Appendix C

Proton Treatment Centers in the US
As of January 2020

Operating Proton Centers in the U.S.
(Including Date Opened):

1. James M. Slater, M.D. Proton Treatment and Research Center at Loma Linda University Medical Center, Loma Linda, CA (1990)
2. UCSF Medical Center, Davis, CA (low-energy system, treats only ocular tumors), (1994)
3. Francis H. Burr Proton Therapy Center at Massachusetts General Hospital, Boston, MA (2001)
4. M.D. Anderson Cancer Center's Proton Center, Houston, TX (2006)
5. University of Florida Health Proton Therapy Institute, Jacksonville, FL (2006)
6. Oklahoma Proton Center, Oklahoma City, OK (2009)
7. Northwestern Medicine Chicago Proton Center, Chicago, IL (2010)
8. Hampton University Proton Therapy Institute, Hampton, VA (2010)
9. Roberts Proton Therapy Center at UPENN, Philadelphia, PA (2010)
10. ProCure Proton Therapy Center, NJ/Metro NY, Somerset, NJ (2012)
11. SCCA Proton Therapy Center, Seattle, WA (2013)
12. S. Lee Kling Proton Therapy Center at Barnes-Jewish Hospital, St. Louis, MO (2013)
13. Provision CARES Proton Therapy, Knoxville, TN (2014)
14. California Protons Cancer Therapy Center, San Diego, CA (2014)

15. Willis-Knighton Proton Therapy Center, Shreveport, LA (2014)
16. Ackerman Cancer Center, Jacksonville, FL (2015)
17. Laurie Proton Center of Robert Wood Johnson University Hospital, New Brunswick, NJ (2015)
18. Texas Center for Proton Therapy, Irving/Dallas, TX (2015)
19. St. Jude Red Frog Events Proton Therapy Center, Memphis, TN (2015)
20. Mayo Clinic Proton Beam Therapy Center, Rochester, MN (2015)
21. Mayo Clinic Proton Beam Therapy Center, Phoenix, AZ (2016)
22. Maryland Proton Treatment Center, Baltimore, MD (2016)
23. Orlando Health Proton Treatment Center, Orlando, FL (2016)
24. University Hospital Seidman Cancer Center, Cleveland OH (2016)
25. Cincinnati Children's Proton Therapy Center, Cincinnati, OH (2016)
26. Beaumont Health Proton Therapy Center, Detroit, MI (2017)
27. Baptist Hospital Cancer Institute PTC, Miami, FL (2017)
28. Medstar Georgetown University Hospital PTC, Washington, DC (2018)
29. Emory Proton Therapy Center, Atlanta, GA (2018)
30. Provision CARES Proton Therapy, Nashville, TN (2018)
31. Stephensen Cancer Center, Oklahoma City, OK (2019)
32. McLaren Proton Therapy Center, Flint, MI (2019)
33. Johns Hopkins Sibley Memorial Hospital, Washington, DC (2019)
34. UAB Medicine, Univ. of Alabama, Birmingham (2020)

Note: There are many more proton centers in the U.S. that are under construction or in the design or planning stage. For a complete listing of proton centers worldwide, visit the Particle Therapy Co-Operative Group (PTCOG) website

Appendix D

References

Book References

American Cancer Society, *American Cancer Society's Complete Guide to Prostate Cancer*

Campbell Ph.D., T. Colin, *The China Study*

Centeno, Arthur, Onik, Gary, Kusler, Jack Allen, *Prostate Cancer – A Patient's Guide to Treatment*

Clapp, Ph.D., J.D., *Prostate Health in 90 Days*

Diehl, DrHSc, MPH, Hans & Ludington, MSD, Aileen, *Health Power – Health by Choice Not Chance*

Ellsworth, M.D., Pamela, 100 *Questions & Answers about Prostate Cancer*

Farrington, Thomas, *Battling the Killer Within and Winning*

Groopman, M.D., Jerome, *How Doctors Think*

Harter-Pierce, Tanya, *Outsmart Your Cancer*

Hennenfent, M.D., Bradley, *Surviving Prostate Cancer without Surgery*

Kaltenbach, Don, with Tim Richards, *Prostate Cancer, A Survivor's Guide*

Katz, M.D., Aaron E., *Dr. Katz's Guide to Prostate Health*

Lange, Paul H., and Adamec, Christine, *Prostate Cancer for Dummies*

Lawrenson, Alan G., *An ABC of Prostate Cancer in 2015*

Lyon Howe, Desiree, *His Prostate and Me*

Marks, M.D., Sheldon, *Prostate and Cancer, A Family Guide to Diagnosis, Treatment and Survival.*

Myers, M.D., Charles "Snuffy," *Beating Prostate Cancer: Hormonal Therapy and Diet*

Myers, M.D., Charles "Snuffy," *The New Prostate Cancer Nutrition Book*

Nelson, Ron, *Protons versus Prostate Cancer Exposed*

Priest, James D., *Beating Prostate Cancer without Surgery*

Ricketts, David, *Eat to Beat Prostate Cancer Cookbook*

Sandage, Stanley, *He Said, 'You Have Prostate Cancer'*

Servan-Schreiber, M.D., Ph.D., *Anti Cancer a New Way of Life*

Scholz, M.D., Mark, *The Key to Prostate Cancer*

Strum, M.D., Stephen and Pogliano, Donna, *A Primer on Prostate Cancer*

Todd, Laurie, *Fight Your Health Insurer and Win*

Wallner, Kent, *Prostate Cancer – A Non-Surgical Perspective*

Walsh, M.D., Patrick, *The Prostate: A Guide for Men and the Women Who Love Them*

Other References:

A Contemporary Prostate Cancer Grading System: A Validated Alternative to the Gleason Score. Eur Urol (2015), Epstein JI, Zelefsky MJ, Sjoberg DD, et al.

About.com's Guide to Prostate Cancer, Matthew Schmitz, M.D.

Clinical Applications of Proton Radiation Treatment at Loma Linda University: Review of a Fifteen-Year Experience, Jerry D. Slater, M.D. Technology in Cancer Research and Treatment, Vol. 5, No. 2, April 2006.

Clinical Correlates to PSA Spikes and Positive Repeat Biopsies after Prostate Brachytherapy, Urology 62:683-688, 2003.

Comparative Effectiveness of Proton vs Proton Therapy as Part of Concurrent Chemoradiotherapy for Locally Advanced Cancer, Brian James M. Metz, MD et. al., JAMA Oncology, Nov. 25, 2019

Comparison of Conventional-Dose v. High-Dose Conformal Radiation Therapy in Clinically Localized Adenocarcinoma of the Prostate, Anthony Zietman, M.D., Jerry D. Slater, M.D., Carl Rossi, M.D. et. al. Journal of the American Medical Association, Vol. 294, No. 10, Sept. 14, 2005

Conformal Proton Beam Radiotherapy of Cancer, Carl J. Rossi, Jr., MD, Department of Radiation Medicine, Loma Linda University Medical Center, Loma Linda, CA, March 5, 1996

Conformal Proton Beam Radiation Therapy for Prostate Cancer. Carl J. Rossi, Jr., M.D. Prostate Cancer Communication Newsletter, Vol. 33, No. 1, March 2007

Considering Radiation for Prostate Cancer, Johns Hopkins Medical Letter. Vol. 17, Issue 6, August 2005

Curing Prostate Cancer, Forbes. Nov. 1, 2004

Developing and Understanding a Hospital-based Proton Facility: Bringing Physics to Medicine, James M. Slater, M.D. Technology in Cancer Research and Treatment ISSN 1533-0346, Vol. 6, No. 4 Supplement, August 2007.

Filling a Research Gap. – Study focusing on black men shows value of prostate cancer screening in midlife. Harvard Medical School, News & Research, Oct. 17, 2018

Getting a Second Opinion on Your Pathology Report, Cancer ABCs, 2018, https://www.cancerabcs.org/pathology-2nd-opinions

Gleason score 2-4 adenocarcinoma of the prostate on needle biopsy: A diagnosis that should not be made, Jonathan Epstein, M.D., Amer. Journal of Surgical Pathology, 2000, Oct. 24 (10): 1443-4

Impotence Following Radical Prostatectomy: Insight into Etiology and Prevention, PC Walsh, PJ Donker, J Urol. February 2017: S165-S170

Incidence of second malignancies among patients treated with proton versus photon radiation, Chung CS, Yock TI, Nelson K, et al., *Int J Radiat Oncol Biol Phys* 2013 Sept. 1;87(1):46-52

Interpreting a Pathology Report: 15 Biopsy and Gleason Questions Answered by a Leading Pathologist, Jonathan Epstein, MD, Prostate Cancer Research Institute, Feb. 1, 2016

Is Robotic Prostate Cancer Surgery Bad Health Advice? Bert Vorstman, BSc, MD, MS, FAAP, FRACS, FACS, UrologyWeb.com, June 10, 2019.

Laparoscopic radical prostatectomy: perioperative complications in an initial and consecutive series of 80 cases, Eur Urol. 2003 Aug;44(2):190-4

Natural history of progression after PSA elevation following radical prostatectomy, Journal of the American Medical Association. 281(17):1591-1597, 1999 C.R. Pound, et al.

Novel Approaches May Decrease Prostate Biopsy Infection Risk, John Schieszer, *Renal & Urology News,* May 1, 2018

The Promise of Proton Therapy is Two-Fold – Less Toxicity and Higher Cure Rates Than Achievable with X-ray Therapy. Nancy Price Mendenhall, MD
http://oi.accc-cancer.org/articles/mayjune07/mendelhall.pdf

Prostate Biopsy Procedure Eliminates Risk of Infection, Betty Olt, Northwell Health, Sept. 7, 2018,
https://www.northwell.edu/news/prostate-biopsy-procedure-eliminates-risk-of-infection-0

Prostate Cancer Specific Survival Following Salvage Radiotherapy vs. Observation in Men with Biochemical Recurrence After Radical Prostatectomy, JAMA, June 18, 2008 – Vol. 299, No. 23, Patrick Walsh, M.D., et al.

Prostate Cancer Tests Might Miss One In Seven Cases, Daily University Science News July 2001

Prostate Cancer Treatment – Deception and Lies, Bert Vorstman, BSc, MD, MS, FAAP, FRACS, FACS, UrologyWeb.com, Feb. 21, 2019.

Prostate Health – Early Detection, Informed Choices, Mayo Clinic Health Letter, June 2005.

Prostate-specific antigen doubling times in patients who have failed radical prostatectomy-correlation with histologic characteristics of the primary cancer, Urology. 49:737-742, 1997 R.S. Pruthi, et al.

Proton Therapy for Prostate Cancer – The Initial Loma Linda Experience, Journal of Radiation Oncology, Biology, Physics Vol. 59, No. 2, pp 348-352, 2004

PSA Threshold for Prostate Cancer Misses a 'Significant' Number of Cancers, J Urol 2001;165:757-760

343

Radiation Therapy for Prostate Cancer – When is Radiation Therapy Used? American Cancer Society,
https://www.cancer.org/cancer/prostate-cancer/treating/radiation-therapy.html

Regrets after Prostate Surgery, Tara Parker-Pope, *New York Times*, Aug. 27, 2008

Role of Active Surveillance in the Management of Men with Localized Prostate Cancer. NIH State-of-the-Science Conference, Dec. 5-7, 2011

The Patient Proton, LeRoy Butler, PhD, Professor of Organic Chemistry, Norwich University

Screening Rectal Culture to Identify Fluoroquinolone-resistant Organisms Before Transrectal Prostate Biopsy, Urology. 2013 Jul; 82(1): 67-71. Doi: 10.1016/j.urology.2013.02.068

The Secrets of Long Life, National Geographic, November 2005

Ten Important Questions to Ask if You're Diagnosed with Prostate Cancer, Naeem Rahman, MD, The Washington Post, Health & Science, Jan. 5, 2019

Three Different Anesthesia Techniques for a Comfortable Prostate Biopsy, Urol Ann. 2015 Jul-Sep; 7(3): 339–344. doi: 10.4103/0974-7796.152014

The Treatment of Recurrent Prostate Cancer, Communications Newsletter, Vol. 15, No. 4, Oct. 1999, Charles E. "Snuffy" Myers, M.D.

Transperineal 3D mapping biopsy of the prostate: An essential tool in selecting patients for focal prostate cancer therapy, Urologic Oncology, Vol. 26, Issue 5, pp 506-510 (Sept. 2008)

To Screen or Not to Screen. The Controversy Over Prostate Cancer. Laboratory Medicine V29, No. 8.

344

Variations in Morbidity After Radical Prostatectomy, Colin B. Begg, Peter T. Scardino, M.D., et. al. The New England Journal of Medicine, Vol. 346, No. 15, April 11, 2002.

Vitamin D3 & Slow Growing Recurrent Disease, Prostate Forum, Vol. 10, No. 7, May 2008, Charles "Snuffy" Myers, M.D.

Appendix E
Helpful Prostate Cancer Websites

Ackerman Cancer Center, Jacksonville, FL

https://www.ackermancancercenter.com/

American Cancer Society

www.cancer.org

Baptist Hospital Cancer Institute PTC, Miami, FL

https://baptisthealth.net/cancer-care/treatments-and-services/radiation-therapies/proton-therapy

Beaumont Health Proton Therapy Center, Detroit, MI

https://www.beaumont.org/services/oncology/proton-therapy

Brotherhood of the Balloon

www.protonbob.com

California Protons Cancer Therapy Center, San Diego, CA

https://www.californiaprotons.com

Cancer Care

https://www.cancercare.org/diagnosis/prostate_cancer

Cincinnati Children's Proton Therapy Center, Cincinnati, OH

https://www.uchealth.com/cancer/centers-programs/proton-therapy/

Emory Proton Therapy Center, Atlanta, GA

https://winshipcancer.emory.edu/proton-therapy-center/

Francis H. Burr Proton Therapy Center at Massachusetts General Hospital, Boston, MA

https://www.massgeneral.org/cancer-center/radiation-oncology/treatments-and-services/proton-therapy

Hampton University Proton Therapy Institute, Hampton, VA

http://www.hamptonproton.org/

James M. Slater, MD Proton Treatment & Research Center, Loma Linda Univ. Cancer Center	www.protons.com
Johns Hopkins Sibley Memorial Hospital, Washington DC	https://www.hopkinsmedicine.org/sibley-memorial-hospital/
Kantor & Kantor Law Firm. Relief from insurance denials	https://www.kantorlaw.net/
Laurie Proton Center of Robert Wood Johnson University Hospital, New Brunswick, NJ	https://www.rwjbh.org/rwj-university-hospital-new-brunswick/treatment-care/radiation-oncology/proton-therapy/
Maryland Proton Treatment Center, Baltimore, MD	https://mdproton.com/
Mayo Clinic Proton Beam Therapy Center, Phoenix, AZ	https://www.mayoclinic.org/departments-centers/proton-beam-therapy-program/sections/overview/ovc-20185491
Mayo Clinic Proton Beam Therapy Center, Rochester, MN	https://www.mayoclinic.org/departments-centers/proton-beam-therapy-program/sections/overview/ovc-20185491
McLaren Proton Therapy Center, Flint, MI	https://www.karmanos.org/karmanos/proton-therapy-center
M.D. Anderson Cancer Center's Proton Center, Houston, TX	https://www.mdanderson.org/patients-family/diagnosis-treatment/care-centers-clinics/proton-therapy-center.html

Medstar Georgetown University Hospital PTC, Washington, DC	ps://www.medstargeorgetown.or g/our-services/cancer-care/treatments/proton-therapy-center/
MedicineNet	https://www.medicinenet.com/pr ostate_cancer/article.htm
MedlinePlus	https://medlineplus.gov/prostate cancer.html
Memorial Sloan Kettering Prostate Cancer Cure Rate Prediction Tool (Nomogram)	https://www.mskcc.org/nomogra ms/prostate/psa_doubling_time
National Association for Proton Therapy	www.proton-therapy.org
NIH National Cancer Institute	https://www.cancer.gov/types/pr ostate
Northwestern Medicine Chicago Proton Center, Chicago, IL	https://www.protoncenter.nm.org
Oklahoma Proton Center, Oklahoma City, OK	https://www.okcproton.com/
OncoLink	https://www.oncolink.org/
Orlando Health Proton Treatment Center, Orlando, FL	https://www.orlandohealthcance r.com/centers/proton-therapy-center
Particle Therapy Co-Operative Group	https://www.ptcog.ch/
Partin Tables, Johns Hopkins Medicine	https://www.hopkinsmedicine.or g/brady-urology-institute/specialties/conditions-and-treatments/prostate-cancer/fighting-prostate-cancer/partin-table.html
Patient Insurance advocacy	www.patientadvocate.org

Phoenix 5 Glossary of Terms	www.phoenix5.org/glossary/glossary.html
ProCure Proton Therapy Center, NJ/Metro NY, Somerset, NJ	https://www.procure.com/
Prostate Cancer Blogs	https://www.healthline.com/health/prostate-cancer/best-blogs-of-the-year#1
Prostate Cancer Foundation	www.prostatecancerfoundation.org
Prostate Cancer Glossary	https://www.webmd.com/prostate-cancer/guide/prostate-cancer-glossary#1
Prostate Cancer Research Institute (PCRI)	www.prostate-cancer.org
Prostate Cancer Wikipedia	https://en.wikipedia.org/wiki/Prostate_cancer
Provision CARES Proton Therapy, Knoxville, TN	https://provisionhealthcare.com/locations-2/knoxville/?utm_source=GMB&utm_medium=organic
Provision CARES Proton Therapy, Nashville, TN	https://provisionhealthcare.com/?utm_source=GMB&utm_medium=Organic
Roberts Proton Therapy Center at UPENN, Philadelphia, PA	https://www.pennmedicine.org/cancer/navigating-cancer-care/programs-and-centers/roberts-proton-therapy-center
SCCA Proton Therapy Center, Seattle, WA	https://www.sccaprotontherapy.com/

S. Lee Kling Proton Therapy Center at Barnes-Jewish Hospital, St. Louis, MO	https://siteman.wustl.edu/treatment/siteman-approach/radiation/proton-beam-therapy/
Stephensen Cancer Center, Oklahoma City, OK	https://stephensoncancercenter.org/
St. Jude Red Frog Events Proton Therapy Center, Memphis, TN	https://www.stjude.org/treatment/services/radiation-oncology/proton-therapy.html
Texas Center for Proton Therapy, Irving/Dallas, TX	https://www.texascenterforprotontherapy.com/
UAB Medicine Proton Center, Univ. of Alabama, Birmingham	https://www.uab.edu/home/
University Hospital Seidman Cancer Center, Cleveland, OH	https://www.uhhospitals.org/locations/uh-seidman-cancer-center
University of Florida Health Proton Therapy Institute, Jacksonville, FL	https://www.floridaproton.org
Us Too Support	www.ustoo.com
Willis-Knighton Proton Therapy Center, Sheveport, LA	https://www.wkhs.com/cancer/cancer-treatment-services/proton-therapy
You Are Not Alone	www.yananow.net

351

Appendix F

Premier Pathology Labs in the U.S.

For Second Opinion on Biopsy Pathology Slides

Jonathan Epstein   410-955-5043
Johns Hopkins Hospital   410-614-6330
Baltimore, MD

David Bostwick, M.D. M.B.A.   800-214-6628
Bostwick Laboratories, Glen Allen, VA

Dianon Laboratories   800-328-2666
Stratford, CT

Index

To arrange media interviews, personal appearances,
or special assistance the author may be able to provide,
send an email to Deb Hickey at

DHickey@protonbob.com

~

To order

You Can Beat Prostate Cancer

by Robert J. Marckini

in bulk quantities (50 to 1,000 copies or more)
send an email to: DHickey@protonbob.com

Books are printed to order, and discounts
are based on order size

Made in the USA
Monee, IL
14 June 2021